Sociology and Nursing Practice Series

Davina Allen and David Hughes
Nursing and the Division of Labour in Healthcare

Lorraine Culley and Simon Dyson
Ethnicity and Nursing Practice

Elaine Denny and Sarah Earle
The Sociology of Long Term Conditions and Nursing Practice

Paul Godin
Risk and Nursing Practice

Margaret Miers
Class, Inequalities and Nursing Practice

Margaret Miers
Gender Issues and Nursing Practice

Sam Porter
Social Theory and Nursing Practice

Geoff Wilkinson and Margaret Miers
Power and Nursing Practice

T024885

Sociology and Nursing Practice Series
Series Standing Order: ISBN 0–333–69329–9
(outside North America only)

You can receive future titles in this series as they are published by placing a standing order.
Please contact your bookseller or, in case of difficulty, write to us at the address below with
your name and address, the title of the series and the ISBN quoted above.

Customer Services Department, Macmillan Distribution Ltd, Houndmills, Basingstoke,
Hampshire RG21 6XS, England

Also by Elaine Denny

E. Denny & S. Earle (eds) (2005) *Sociology for Nurses, Polity,* Cambridge

Also by Sarah Earle

S. Earle, C.E. Lloyd, M. Sidell & S. Spurr (eds) (2007)
Theory and Research in Promoting Public Health, Sage/Open University, London/Milton Keynes

C.E. Lloyd, S. Handsley, J. Douglas, S. Earle & S. Spurr (eds) (2007)
Policy and Practice in Promoting Public Health, Sage/Open University, London/Milton Keynes

J. Douglas, S. Earle, S. Handsley, C.E. Lloyd & S. Spurr (eds) (2007)
A Reader in Promoting Public Health: Challenge and Controversy, Sage/Open University, London/Milton Keynes

S. Earle & K. Sharp (2007)
Sex in Cyberspace: Men Who Pay for Sex, Ashgate, Aldershot

E. Denny & S. Earle (eds) (2005)
Sociology for Nurses, Polity, Cambridge

S. Earle & G. Letherby (eds) (2003)
Gender, Identity and Reproduction: Social Perspectives, Palgrave, Basingstoke

The Sociology of Long Term Conditions and Nursing Practice

Edited by

Elaine Denny

Sarah Earle

palgrave
macmillan

First published 2009 by
PALGRAVE MACMILLAN

Palgrave Macmillan in the UK is an imprint of Macmillan Publishers Limited, registered in England, company number 785998, of Houndmills, Basingstoke, Hampshire RG21 6XS.

Palgrave Macmillan in the US is a division of St Martin's Press LLC, 175 Fifth Avenue, New York, NY 10010.

Palgrave Macmillan is the global academic imprint of the above companies and has companies and representatives throughout the world.

Palgrave® and Macmillan® are registered trademarks in the United States, the United Kingdom, Europe and other countries.

ISBN-13: 978-0-230-51646-5 paperback
ISBN-10: 0-230-51646-7 paperback

This book is printed on paper suitable for recycling and made from fully managed and sustained forest sources. Logging, pulping and manufacturing processes are expected to conform to the environmental regulations of the country of origin.

A catalogue record for this book is available from the British Library.

10 9 8 7 6 5 4 3 2 1
18 17 16 15 14 13 12 11 10 09

Printed and bound in China

Contents

Tables and figures

Series Editors' Preface

It is widely accepted that sociology has the potential to make a significant contribution to nursing's knowledge base. As a discipline, it offers valuable and pertinent insights into the causes and distribution of ill health, the experience of health, illness and disability, the dynamics of health care encounters and the possibilities and limitations of professional care. Equally important, sociology's emphasis on critical reflection encourages nurses to be questioning and self aware, thus helping them to provide flexible, non discriminatory, user-centred care in various situations.

In addition, nursing has long been a noteworthy subject for sociological study, both as a developing and changing profession and as an interactive activity between individuals. Sociologists can struggle, however, to offer insights concerning the actual work that nurses do. This is partially due to the limitations of sociological surveillance. Nurses work in confidential, private and intimate settings with their clients. Sociologists' access to such settings is necessarily restrictive. Moreover, nurses can find it difficult to talk about their work, except, perhaps, to other nurses.

Nursing has a long tradition of drawing on sociology to explore social interaction, particularly to understand social processes such as labelling and stigma. Nurse researchers increasingly draw on social science literature to illuminate the restraints and enablements imposed on individual health care interactions by social structures. Nurses and sociologists work together in multidisciplinary research teams to explore the complexity and dynamics of health and social care policy and practice. This is particularly the case in relation to the experience and management of long term conditions.

The aim of the *Sociology and Nursing Practice Series* is to support links between the disciplines and to increase nursing and sociology's mutual understanding. The authors of the series' titles and chapters have an intimate understanding of nursing and a commitment to a sociological outlook that asserts the salience of wider social forces to the work of nurses. The texts apply sociological theories and concepts to practical aspects of nursing. By concentrating on specific concepts and drawing on research informed by social theory and methods, each book is able to provide the reader with a deeper understanding of the social construction of nurses' work and the experience of health and illness.

The Sociology of Long-term Conditions and Nursing Practice more than fulfils the aims of the book series. We hope reading this book will encourage nurses to analyse critically their practice and profession and to develop their own contribution to enhancing the experience and quality of care.

Margaret Miers, Sam Porter, Geoff Wilkinson

Acknowledgements

Chapter 2

Figure 2.1 is reprinted with permission from Crown copyright with the permission of the controller of HMSO and the Queen's Printer of Scotland.

Figure 2.2 is reprinted with permission from Crown copyright with the permission of the controller of HMSO and the Queen's Printer of Scotland.

Chapter 6

Figure 6.1 is reproduced with permission from National Institute for Health and Clinical Excellence (NICE) (2007) CG023 Depression (amended): management of depression in primary and secondary care. London: NICE. Available from www.nice.org.uk/GG023.

Table 6.1 is reprinted with permission from the American Diabetes Association.

Every effort has been made to trace and acknowledge copyrighted material, but if any items have been accidently overlooked the publisher will be happy to rectify this as quickly as possible.

Contributors

David Cox has been Chair of South Birmingham PCT since April 2002 and was recently re-appointed. He is a member of Birmingham's Health and Well-Being Partnership Committee and has led work on Health and Care Skills and Race Equality in Birmingham and Solihull's health economy. He is a long-standing member of the Board and Trustee of BRAP. Previously, David was a Primary Care Group lay member and Chair of South Birmingham Community Health Council. David is a sociologist and also worked for the University of Central England (previously Birmingham Polytechnic) from 1970 until 2007 retiring from the post of Associate Dean in the Faculty of Health. He is Emeritus Professor of the renamed Birmingham City University.

Elaine Denny is Professor of Health Sociology and Head of Division, Health Policy and Public Health at Birmingham City University. She has a background in hospital and community nursing and taught health sociology to students on health related courses for 20 years. Her research interests focus around women as recipients and providers of health care, and she has published work on women's experience of IVF (in vitro fertilization), the experience of endometriosis, and on the occupation of nursing. Elaine has co-authored with Sarah Earle a health sociology text *Sociology for Nurses*. Her current research is a Research for Patient Benefit funded collaborative study on endometriosis and cultural diversity aimed at improving services for minority ethnic women. She is also involved in assessing the patient perspective in a number of NIHR funded clinical trials in collaboration with Birmingham Women's Hospital where she is Honorary Research Associate.

Sarah Earle is Senior Lecturer in Health and Social Care at the Open University. She was involved in the production of the popular third-level Open University Course, *K311: Promoting*

Public Health: Skills, Perspectives and Practice and the co-publication of the following associated texts: S. Earle, C.E. Lloyd, M. Sidell and S. Spurr (eds) (2007) *Theory and Research in Promoting Public Health*, Sage/Open University; C.E. Lloyd, S. Handsley, J. Douglas, S. Earle and S. Spurr (eds) (2007) *Policy and Practice in Promoting Public Health*, Sage/Open University; and J. Douglas, S. Earle, S. Handsley, C.E. Lloyd and S. Spurr (eds) (2007) *A Reader in Promoting Public Health: Challenge and Controversy*, Sage/Open University. She is particularly interested in reproductive and sexual health and has published widely in this area. For example, see: S. Earle and K. Sharp (2007), *Sex in Cyberspace: Men Who Pay for Sex*, Ashgate; S. Earle and G. Letherby (2007) 'Conceiving time? Experiences of women who do or do not conceive', *Sociology of Health and Illness*, Vol. 29 (2), pp. 233–50; S. Earle and G. Letherby (eds) (2003) *Gender, Identity and Reproduction: Social Perspectives*, Palgrave. She is also Convenor of the British Sociological Association's Human Reproduction Study Group and Chair of the Open University's Birth and Death Research Group. Sarah is interested in the application of sociology to health care education and practice. Her publications in this area include: S. Church and S. Earle (2006) 'Approaches to sociology within midwifery education', *British Journal of Midwifery*, Vol. 14 (6), 01 June, pp. 342–345; E. Denny and S. Earle (eds) (2005) *Sociology for Nurses*, Polity; and, S. Earle (2001), 'Teaching sociology within the speech and language therapy curriculum', *Education for Health: Change in Training and Practice*, Vol. 14 (3), November, pp. 383–391.

Tom Heller is a General Practitioner in a deprived area of North Sheffield. For the last 20 years he has been Senior Lecturer in Health Studies at the Faculty of Health and Social Care at the Open University. He has been involved in writing a number of undergraduate courses and producing multi-media teaching materials. His clinical practice currently includes some innovative methods of COPD rehabilitation using various group-based activities.

Alistair Hewison has a background in nursing, working as Staff Nurse, Charge Nurse and Nurse Manager in the NHS in Birmingham, Oxford and Warwickshire. He is now Head of the

School of Health Sciences at the University of Birmingham. His areas of teaching centre around the management and organization of health care. Research interests include change in health care, nursing management and nursing policy. He is author of *Management for Nurses and Health Professionals* (Blackwell 2004) and is currently working on a forthcoming book *Policy and Policy Analysis for Nurses* (Wiley-Blackwell). He is also Associate Editor of the *Journal of Nursing Management.*

Gayle Letherby is Professor of Sociology at the University of Plymouth. Her research and writing interests are varied and include reproductive and non-parental identities, working and learning in higher education and the sociology of travel and transport. In addition throughout her career she has been interested in all things methodological. Key publications include G. Letherby (2003) *Feminist Research in Theory and Practice,* Open University Press; and G. Letherby and P. Bywaters (2007) *Extending Social Research: Application, Implementation and Publication,* Open University Press.

Cathy E. Lloyd is Senior Lecturer in the Faculty of Health and Social Care at the Open University. In 1991, after gaining her PhD in community medicine (Public Health) at the University of London, Dr Lloyd moved to the United States where she coordinated a longitudinal study on the natural history of type 1 diabetes. She then gained an R.D. Lawrence Fellowship from Diabetes UK and went on to study the impact of stress on diabetes. She has been with the Open University since 1998, teaching second and third level courses on health, diabetes care, and public health. In 2003 she received a teaching award for her work on the pre-registration nursing programme. Her current research includes a study of the experiences of pregnancy and childbirth in women with diabetes, and investigating fear of hypoglycaemia in children and young people with diabetes. In collaboration with De Montfort, Leicester and Warwick Universities, she is also developing alternative modes of data collection for people whose main language is spoken and not written. With more than 70 publications to her credit, Dr Lloyd has written and taught extensively on psychological factors and diabetes. She is currently Associate Editor of the journal, *Diabetic Medicine.*

Lesley Lockyer qualified as a State Registered Nurse in 1980 followed by a BSc (Hons) in Nursing Studies in 1987 and an MSc in Social Research in 1991. Lesley's clinical career was spent working in Intensive Care Units and Cardiac Units in London, Guildford and Exeter. From 1990 Lesley worked as a research nurse at the Royal Brompton and Harefield Hospital NHS trust and it was during this time that she developed an interest in women's experience of coronary heart disease which led to her PhD in Medical Sociology completed in 2000 from Royal Holloway College, University of London and entitled 'The Experience of Women in the Diagnosis and Treatment of Coronary Heart Disease'. After a post doctoral research fellowship in Cardiac Nursing at the University of Leeds Lesley moved in 2002 to the University of the West of England, Bristol as Senior Lecturer teaching research methods and latterly the sociology of health and illness in the Faculty of Health and Life Sciences. Lesley continues to write and research around coronary heart disease. Her other research interests include the sociology of nursing work, learning and teaching. Recent research topics have included witnessed resuscitation by family members; a comparison of emergency nurses, emergency nurse practitioners and emergency care practitioners' clinical reasoning and decision making in managing patients presenting with chest pain; and a survey of paramedics' perceptions of their role in giving thrombolytic treatment for acute ST segment elevation myocardial infarction.

Ann Mitchell is Lecturer and Mental Health Lead for the pre-registration nursing course at the Open University. She is an experienced Community Mental Health Nurse with 20 years experience in designing, managing and leading undergraduate courses and postgraduate modules. These covered a range of health courses including community nursing and mental health. She developed strong clinical links with mentors and assessors in the local Trust's practice settings. Through a managerial secondment she led and implemented clinical governance principles and mental health policies and strategies within a community mental health Trust. Her current research interests include the physical and mental health needs of black and minority ethnic groups in a multi-cultural society. She has contributed to a number of publications. Her recent writing includes a chapter on stigma, discrimination and ethnicity and a co-authored research article on the mental health role of practice nurses in primary care. Ann has been invited to present conference papers both nationally and internationally, the most recent at the Institute of Commonwealth Studies, University of London on 'Migration and health in Guyanese women'. Other key international activities that she has participated in are lecturer exchange visits to Sweden, Finland and New York. Ann is also an active trustee of the International Institute of Child and Adolescent Mental Health, a charity that organizes and delivers mental health conferences in the United Kingdom and study tours to lesser developed countries.

Erica Richardson has an academic background in the disciplines of health promotion and Russian studies, and the main focus of her postgraduate studies looked at the development of health promotion in the Russian Federation, particularly in the areas of drug and alcohol use. It is through her research examining the role of non-government organizations in the provision of services for injecting drug users that she became involved in European Commission funded projects working both on support for people living with HIV/AIDS across Europe and on HIV/AIDS prevention in Central and Eastern Europe. On completing her PhD in 2002, Erica worked on the ESRC funded project ' "Everyday" but not "normal": drug use and youth cultural practice in Russia' at the University of Birmingham, where she still holds an honorary fellowship in the Centre for Russian and East European Studies (CREES). After briefly working as Research Fellow in the School of Health and Related Research (ScHARR) at the University of Sheffield, Erica joined the European Centre for Health of Societies in Transition (ECOHOST) at the London School of Hygiene and Tropical Medicine in October 2005. She is currently conducting research on the development of health systems and policies in countries of the former Soviet Union and Mongolia; examining different approaches to the organization, financing and delivery of health services as well as describing the institutional framework, process, content and implementation of health policies.

Pauline Savy is a sociologist at the Albury-Wodonga Campus of La Trobe University, Australia. Pauline's doctoral thesis is an ethnographic study of the problem of self-identity in dementia. Her interests, stemming from this research, include exploring methodologies for capturing the experiences of individuals who cannot give conventionally coherent accounts of themselves. Prior to taking up a career in sociology, Pauline held clinical, administrative and educational positions in the fields of aged care and psychiatric nursing. Publications include: B. Furze, P. Savy, R. Brym, and J. Lie (in press) *Sociology in Today's World*, Melbourne, Thomson; P. Savy (guest ed.) (2005) 'Closing Asylums for the mentally ill: Social consequences', *Health Sociology Review*, Vol. 14 (3), pp. 205–214; P. Savy (2005) 'Outcry and silence: the social implications of asylum closure', *Health Sociology Review*, Vol. 14 (3), pp. 215–229; K. Richmond and P. Savy (2005) 'In sight, in mind: mental health policy and the deinstitutionalization of psychiatric hospitals', *Health Sociology Review*, Vol. 14: 3; P. Savy and A. Sawyer (2007) 'Risk, suffering and competing narratives in the psychiatric assessment of an Iraqi refugee', *Culture Medicine and Psychiatry* (2008).

Timothy Chas Skinner is Associate Professor at the CUCRH, Geraldton, Western Australia. After a background in residential social work with young offenders he trained as a psychologist at the University of Westminster and University of Surrey. Following on from his PhD studies in adolescents with type 1 diabetes, he has developed an extensive track record of research in both type 1 and type 2 diabetes, including the development of interventions and health care professional training. This includes 50 peer reviewed publications, eight book chapters, three National Awards, two International Awards, and over £2.5million in collaborative research awards. He is a former Associate Editor of *Diabetic Medicine*, and co-editor of the book *Psychology and Diabetes Care*.

Jonathan Tritter is Chief Executive of the recently established NHS Centre for Involvement and Professorial Fellow in the Institute of Governance and Public Management, Warwick Business School. After completing degrees at the University of Chicago and a doctorate at Oxford University he spent three years as a postdoctoral research fellow at the Social Sciences Research Centre at South Bank University before joining the University of Warwick in 1995. Being the author of more than 50 publications, his main research interests relate to public participation and lay experience in health and policy making particularly in relation to cancer, mental health and environmental policy. He is Docent at the Department of Sociology, University of Helsinki, Visiting Senior Research Fellow at the Finnish National Research and Development Centre for Welfare and Health and Visiting Professor at the Finnish Environment Institute, Research Policy Program. As Associate Director of the University of Warwick, Institute of Health, he coordinates the User/University Teaching and Research Action Partnership in Health and Social Care which supports user involvement in research and teaching across the University.

His recent publications include: E. Anderson, J. Tritter and R. Wilson (eds) (2006) *Healthy Democracy: Involving People in Health and Social Care*. London: INVOLVE; J. Tritter and A. McCallum (2006) 'The Snakes and Ladders of User Involvement: Moving beyond Arnstein', *Health Policy*. Vol. 76 (2), pp. 156–168; H.E. Lester, J. Tritter and H. Sorohan (2005) 'Providing "good enough" primary care for people with serious mental illness – a focus group study', *British Medical Journal*, Vol. 330, pp. 1122–1127; and J. Tritter, N. Daykin, S. Evans and M. Sanidas (2003) *Improving Cancer Services through User Involvement*. Oxford: Radcliffe Medical Press.

Introduction

Elaine Denny and Sarah Earle

It is a frequently repeated saying that people are living longer, yet living at least some of those extra years in poor health. The reasons for this longevity are mainly the result of environmental factors such as improved living standards, a cleaner environment and better nutrition resulting in a reduction in the major causes of mortality of previous eras. Yet it is not just older people who are surviving illness that would have proved fatal in the past. People of working age, children and young people are also living with diseases and following injuries that would have proved fatal as recently as one generation ago. Diseases such as cancer and HIV, which used to be considered a death sentence and survivors being thought of as incredibly lucky, are now being managed for many years, with those affected being able to live a life that can range from near normal to severely incapacitated. Similarly, premature birth was frequently followed by premature death, but now neonatal care means that many of these babies survive. However, predictions about how much, if any, disability such children will experience are difficult to make. So improvements in survival are making new demands on the health care professionals who work with those affected by long term illness and disability; and nurses are in the vanguard of attempting to address them.

Those people with multiple conditions are disproportionate users of health services. People with long term conditions visit their General Practitioner (GP) more frequently, experience more hospital admissions and stay in hospital longer than the rest of the population (Wilson, Buck and Ham, 2005). A high proportion of emergency hospital admissions and of total bed days are for exacerbations of long term illness (DH, 2004). The major health concern of the twenty first century, therefore, is not the acute illnesses which the NHS and most Western health care systems were set up to deal with, but the management and improvement of the quality of life for those living with a condition or disease for which there is no cure. The policy challenge is to move away from a health care system based around acute episodes of ill health to one that supports those with long term illness in appropriate care settings. A further challenge is that long term conditions tend to be disproportionately found in the most disadvantaged sections of society, and a reduction in health inequalities is also necessary in order to reduce their incidence.

From the above discussion we can begin to understand renewed government interest in long term conditions and a move from hospital to primary and community care as the focus of health care. Nurses are pivotal to this move, expanding their roles in areas such as non-medical prescribing and the role of Community Matron. When people are not managed effectively they use physical, emotional, and financial resources that would not be necessary if problems were prevented or diagnosed early. Their own expertise in managing their condition – built up from personal experience – supplemented by the research that many people carry out, is not utilized to the best effect. They are not treated as partners in their care, and their quality of life suffers. It is the recognition of these factors that has focused governments' health agenda on better ways of managing those with long term illness.

Some of these issues have been highlighted by the work of policy analysts and sociologists of health and illness over many years. Raising them here demonstrates that nurses working in this area need more than just their clinical knowledge of the illnesses that they confront. They also need to be able to engage in the debates about the most appropriate delivery of care to their client groups, and to see their work in a broader context. This book utilises classic sociological work and more recent empirical evidence to produce a sociology of long term conditions that reflects the contemporary situation.

In common with other volumes in the *Sociology for Nurses* series this book demonstrates the ways in which a sociological imagination can inform and enhance nursing practice in the context of a changing health service. Nurses are in the forefront of caring for people with long term conditions both in hospital, in the community and other settings; yet most existing text-books focus on the sociology of disability, and are not specifically written for nurses. While acknowledging the importance of this work, this volume places emphasis on the application of the sociology of disability *and* chronic illness to the practice of nursing people with long term conditions. The book is divided into two parts. Part I focuses on theory, policy, and research relating to chronic illness and long term conditions. Part II examines a range of long term conditions exploring how the development of a sociological imagination can enhance nursing practice in this field.

We have in this introduction been using the terms 'chronic illness', 'long term illness', and 'long term conditions' inter-changeably. Partly, this reflects changing terminology over the years. Early work from whatever academic discipline spoke of chronic illness, which was taken to mean long lasting and incurable. This was contrasted with acute illness which was short term, and self limiting or curable. A problem with this term is that for some people for some of the time they are not ill, their condition relapses and goes into remission, but does not go away. 'Chronic' too does not adequately describe something that is characterised by acute flare ups. On the other hand many people are ill for a lot of their lives, they have symptoms that need treatment or some form of health intervention, so 'condition' does not sufficiently reflect their situation. Recent government initiatives have used the term 'long term conditions', for example in the National Service Framework for Long Term Conditions (DH, 2005). Long term conditions are defined on the Department of Health website as those conditions that at present have no cure, but that can be controlled or contained by medication or other interventions. There is not, however, any rationale given for the change to current terminology, nor indication of any dissatisfaction expressed about the continued use of the term chronic illness. Even amongst the authors of this book there has been disagreement over terminology. However, this disagreement has been characterized by a concern for the most appropriate terminology for the particular group of people that the author is writing about. As editors we have left the terminology to the discretion of individual authors within their own chapters, and of course when quoting or citing work the discourse of the original author has been employed. For the title of the book, however, we have decided to adopt the term 'long term conditions' since it most accurately reflects contemporary use, and has the most currency within policy and nursing practice.

References

Department of Health (DH) *The NHS Improvement Plan* (3398) (London: DH, 2004).

Department of Health (DH) *The National Service Framework for long term conditions* (London: DH, 2005).

Wilson, T., Buck D., and Ham C., 'Rising to the challenge: will the NHS support people with long term conditions?', *British Medical Journal*, 330 (2005) 657–661.

I Introduction

Elaine Denny and Sarah Earle

Part I of this volume focuses on theory, policy, and research relating to chronic illness and long term conditions. Using a sociological framework it considers the way in which contemporary perspectives and policies have developed, and examines the influence of research on policy and practice. While it may be tempting for busy practitioners to move straight to the empirical 'real world' research of Part II, a reading of these early chapters will facilitate a deeper and contextualised understanding of the lives of those living with long term conditions and the challenges involved in translating government policy into practice.

The first chapter – written by Elaine Denny and Sarah Earle – takes a historical approach to the development of a sociology of chronic illness, beginning with Parson's concept of the sick role and its applicability to the idea of chronic illness, progressing through some of the major writers in the field up to the very recent post modern perspectives developed by theorists of the sociology of the body. Denny and Earle explain how the genre has moved from exploring specific disease states, thus reinforcing a biomedical model of illness, to one that recognises the diversity of human experience. This chapter provides the theoretical framework which informs the chapters in Part II, and demonstrate how both structural and interpretive sociology have informed research into chronic illness and long term conditions.

Chapter 2 then moves to the policy issues and policy responses provoked by the growing importance of long term conditions as a modern health concern. In this chapter, Alistair

Hewison and David Cox set out the policy problems raised by the increasing number of people living in the community with long term illness and disability in the United Kingdom. They identify the challenge that this poses for policy makers and analyze the government's response in terms of policy strategy and initiatives. Hewison and Cox provide an insight into how the care of people with long term conditions is likely to be manged over the next few years, and particular emphasis is given here to the increasing importance for the role of nurses in dealing with this challenge.

In Chapter 3 Gayle Letherby considers issues of method, methodology and epistemology relevant to researching people with long term conditions. This chapter highlights how the methods we choose and our methodological experience are influenced by the topic under investigation. Furthermore, Letherby argues, the research process itself influences the research product, and this chapter provides an overview of these issues highlighting the political significance of issues of method, methodology and epistemology. The chapter offers advice to anyone contemplating conducting their own social research into long term conditions, but the information contained here is equally valuable to those reading the research of others in order to inform their own practice.

These chapters all have the main aim of providing the context in which developments in the management of long term conditions are taking place, and setting the clinical work of practitioners within a social and policy framework. Social science research is increasingly used to inform the development of policy, and to evaluate its implementation and outcomes. This part of the book provides the background with which to move on to Part II which considers individual conditions, and uses empirical and other research work to explore them from a sociological standpoint.

1 Chronic illness, disability and the politics of health

Elaine Denny and Sarah Earle

Introduction

In many modern societies, individuals are living longer lives, but those lives are not always lived in good health. Chronic illness – which refers to a long-term, sometimes permanent and intractable condition – has seen an 'epidemiological explosion' (May, 2005, p. 16) in societies characterized by industrialization, affluence and wealth. Although not all sociologists agree that there has been an epidemiological explosion in chronic illness (Armstrong, 2005) there is, at least, a strong political and policy imperative to understand the distribution of chronic illness, the experiences of those who live with these conditions, and the impact of this on nurses and other practitioners. Sociologists are interested in studying chronic *illness* rather than *disease* because it shifts the focus away from a paternalistic medical approach to health to one which focuses on subjective, lived experiences as well as on the relationships between patients and practitioners, and between these and the wider society.

Sociologists have been interested in health and healthcare for over 50 years, although there have been developments in conceptual and theoretical, as well as empirical and methodological, emphases over time. Early accounts of illness in the 1950s drew on functionalist sociological theory to develop ideas about the role of sickness within society and on the relationships between doctor and patient. This chapter begins by examining this idea by exploring the work of Talcott Parsons (1951) and his ideas on the 'sick role'.

Later analyses of chronic illness were influenced more by an interpretivist sociological tradition, which sought to understand lived experiences and the ways in which individuals coped with chronic illness in the day-to-day. The work of Erving Goffman (1963) has been particularly influential in developing an understanding of the relationship between stigma and chronic illness and has been applied to a wide range of conditions.

Following on from this, an interest in identity and personal biography developed. This focused on how chronic illness, which is often uncertain and intractable, caused disruption in the lives of those individuals with chronic illness. The work of Michael Bury (1982) and the development of his concept of 'biographical disruption' has been highly influential in this field. Narrative approaches to research on chronic illness then became popular as a method of exploring how individuals make sense of chronic illness.

The trajectory of chronic illness is not only uncertain but it is one that can lead to considerable pain and disability. So, much later, the development of disability theory and the sociology of disability began to challenge some of the conceptual and theoretical ideas on the sociology of chronic illness. Disability theorists were keen to demonstrate how disability should be located within the barriers posed by society rather than located within the body and in relation to specific individual experiences of chronic illness. The social model of disability, which was firstly developed by Mike Oliver (1983), highlights the importance of focusing on the structures of society, rather than on the individual. These ideas have had considerable political, practical and, to some extent, theoretical, currency.

However, most recently, the sociology of the body has sought to bring the body 'back in' to sociological accounts of health, disability and chronic illness, in particular. This approach – whilst accepting the importance of structural perspectives – tries to take into account the reality of living with chronic illness as one in which pain and disability is located within the body itself, and not just in relation to the social structure of society. Drawing on the various theoretical positions briefly outlined above, this chapter provides an overview of changing sociological perspectives on chronic illness.

Doctors, patients and the 'sick role'

The notion of the sick role was developed by Talcott Parsons in the 1950s to explain how the 'deviance' of the sick role is managed. It was already known that the sick person occupies a special position in society but Parsons produced the first systematic sociological study of illness. Parsons (1951) argued that illness is a social phenomenon and needs to be understood in terms of societal functioning and in relation to the cultural values that exist within that society. More specifically, there is a functional interest of society in the minimization of illness, as the interference it causes to normal functioning risks becoming a social deviance unless it is controlled in some way. It is the role of the medical profession to sanction and legitimize illness, but it is the role of the patient that is of more interest to us here. Parsons developed the sick role to explain the conditions under which a person is able to assume the status of 'sick'. There are four aspects to the sick role, usually expressed as two rights and two responsibilities. The rights are that a sick person is exempted from their normal social responsibilities and, as they are not held responsible for their illness, they can expect to be taken care of. The responsibilities of the sick underpin the conditional nature of the rights and are the obligation to want to get well and to seek technically competent help to do so. The medical practitioner too has obligations in this scenario. He/she must act solely in the best interests of the patient – what Parsons calls 'collectivity orientation' (1951, p. 435) – and must work to the highest standards of clinical competence. The rights of the doctor are more difficult to determine (Gerhardt, 1987), but focus on the exclusive access that the medical profession possesses to the body, and to privileged information.

Some sociologists now consider Parsons' work to be outdated and irrelevant, although this is by no means universal (e.g., see Shilling, 2002 or Williams, 2005). In part, this perspective is based on the many critiques of Parsons' work that have emerged over the years. For example, Parsons has been criticized for failing to fully account for differences in age, class, ethnicity and gender in his analyses. The concept of the sick role has also been questioned in relation to how relevant it might be to people with mental health problems. However, among the many critiques of Parsons one of the most consistent has been the failure of the sick role concept to account for chronic and long-term illness, where a cure and return to a pre-illness state is not possible. Gerhardt (1987), however, argues that such criticism is based on an incorrect understanding of Parson's work. Indeed there are pointers within his work that he recognized the diversity of illnesses and the likelihood of recovery. For example: 'First it must be remembered that there is an enormous range of different types of illness and degrees of severity' (Parsons, 1951, p. 440) and: 'The urgency of the need for help will vary with the severity of disability, suffering and risk of death or serious, lengthy or permanent disablement.' (p. 440). In 1974 he made clear his belief that the sick role concept could be applied to chronic illness: 'The issue is one of approximation rather than accomplishment of the goal of recovery, and permanently being exempted from a partial range of one's duties rather than temporarily being exempted from more or less the whole range of one's duties.' (Gerhardt, 1987, p. 119).

Parson's examination of sickness and the role of the patient and the doctor was a structural analysis that focused on the functioning of society, but in the 1960s sociological research moved to a consideration of more individualistic accounts of chronic illness.

Stigma and chronic illness as metaphor

The concept of stigma is generally attributed to the influential work of sociologist Erving Goffman and, in particular, to his book, *Stigma: Notes on the Management of a Spoiled Identity* (1963), although the concept is now also widely used within the social sciences more generally (Scambler, 2006). Goffman describes stigma as a socially constructed phenomenon whereby an individual shows: 'evidence of an attribute that makes him different from others ... and of a less desirable kind ... he is then reduced in our minds from a whole and usual person, to a tainted, discounted one ... whom has a spoiled identity' (Goffman, 1963, p. 12).

Stigma, therefore, refers to the possession of an attribute that is deeply discrediting, setting an individual aside as deviant, rather than as a 'normal' member of society. However, Goffman refers to three distinct types of stigma: first, that which arises from physical deformity; second, that which can be attributed to blemishes of character; and, third, the tribal stigma of race, nation and religion. However, not all stigma are equally discrediting, since some attributes can be hidden from others and others not. Goffman, thus, makes the distinction between discrediting (easily visible) attributes – for example, physical deformity – and discreditable (less visible) attributes – for example, epilepsy. Discrediting attributes are immediately stigmatizing whereas the potential stigma of a discreditable attribute depends upon both the nature of that attribute and the extent to which knowledge of it is contained or managed.

There are many examples in the literature where the concept of stigma has been applied to chronic illness. For example, in a British study of discharge planning within a regional cancer centre (Wilson and Luker, 2006), one of the respondents – Josie (who had undergone palliative surgery for colorectal cancer) – describes her feelings of stigma: 'You feel like you've got a [leper's] bell on you and all that... Don't mention the word. It's like "Don't mention the War!"' (p. 1619). In the same study, another respondent – Dennis – describes his experiences prior to first admission to hospital. In this instance, nobody had actually informed Dennis that he had cancer: 'I had to put two and two together when I came in here to realize that I've got lung cancer... Nobody actually came out with those two words...' (p. 1620). Some of the other potentially adverse affects of being affected by cancer highlighted by this study include dealing with the feelings of close friends and family; this was the respondent Rob's experience who states: '[One] of my closest friends... he can't handle it. He doesn't want to see me until it's all over with. He phoned me every other day. He said "I really can't see you at the moment", which was really weird' (p. 1620). As Goffman notes, the stigmatized individual is often excluded from 'full social acceptance' (1963, p. 9).

Goffman also suggests that there were two distinct sorts of stigma: felt and enacted. Felt stigma relates to the direct experience of negative judgement as a consequence of possessing a discrediting/discreditable attribute, whereas enacted stigma refers to the expectation of such a negative judgement. Some individuals may experience one or both of these types of stigma. An Australian study (Fraser and Treloar, 2006) of people with Hepatitis C – an infection that can lead to chronic illness – illustrates just this point:

> Our interviews indicate that not only do hepatitis C positive people encounter stigmatizing responses from others to whom their health status is usually visible through records – (for example doctors, nurses and other health professionals) – they also grapple with their own feelings of contamination and illegitimacy, that is, with a sense that they carry a hidden stigma that may one day be revealed. (Fraser and Treloar, 2006, p. 102)

Similar experiences of stigma are both felt and enacted by people living with other chronic conditions such as epilepsy (see below) or HIV (Van Brakel, 2006; see also Chapter 8 in this volume).

However, the stigma of living with a chronic condition can not only affect the person with that condition, but it can also affect the people around them. Goffman (1963) refers to this as courtesy stigma, arguing that there is 'a tendency for stigma to spread from the stigmatized individual to his [sic] close connections' and that through these close connections, both individuals are treated 'in some respects as one' and, thus, both stigmatized (p. 30). A review of the impact of courtesy stigma on families of people with mental illness (Corrigan and Miller, 2004) found that family members experienced 'significant discrimination' as a consequence of courtesy stigma (p. 539). Of course, not everyone who associates with people who have chronic conditions experiences this level of stigma. A study of primary caregivers and family members of people living with Alzheimer's disease (Macrae, 1999) found that many did experience courtesy stigma, but certainly not all (see Chapter 9 in this volume).

Some chronic conditions are more stigmatized than others, in particular, when a condition is – correctly or incorrectly – seen to be the consequence of an 'unhealthy' lifestyle. For example, being HIV-positive is often associated with illegal drug-use or promiscuity. Being obese is associated with eating too much and exercising too little (see Chapter 11 in this volume). In other words, a process of victim-blaming can exacerbate feelings and experiences of stigma. A qualitative study of stigma and shame in patients with lung cancer (Chapple, Ziebland and McPherson, 2004), for example, found that respondents (whether they had previously smoked or not) felt unjustly blamed for their condition. The authors of this study conclude that because of a victim-blaming culture, stigma and blame have far reaching consequences for people with lung cancer. The same can be said for people living with many other chronic conditions.

Sontag's work, *Illness and Metaphor* (1979), is also helpful in understanding the meanings society gives to long-term conditions. She argues that certain illnesses, especially those which are poorly understood by society, are ascribed particular meanings. For example, Sontag illustrates how cancer became synonymous with death. That is, illness becomes a metaphor for the problems, fears and anxieties of society. Similarly, being HIV-positive is associated with promiscuity, and obesity is associated with greed, sloth and abundance.

Interpretive perspectives on chronic illness

Much of the interpretive work on chronic illness, including that on stigmatized conditions, emanated from a personal interest (see for example Jobling, 1988; Roth, 1963) and focused on how people with chronic illnesses described the problems they faced and how they coped with them. Jobling (1988), in a multinational study, studied the difference in the knowledge, understanding and evaluation of treatments for psoriasis between health professionals and patients. Psoriasis is a chronic skin complaint that has no cure, so the objective of treatment is containment and a reduction in the appearance of symptoms. The skin is a very visible part of the person and the scaling and flaking of it, characteristic of psoriasis, were associated with uncleanness and consequent shame. As one woman put it: 'I have always felt a sense of shame. I feel it most when I look at my body. I try to hide it even from my friends, especially from friends in fact. But the scales make it difficult. It is such a dirty disease' (Jobling, 1988, p. 230).

Jobling described the treatment rituals involved in living with the disease. For the patient these were as much part of the problem as the solution, but they were taken for granted by dermatologists who were mainly interested in their clinical effectiveness, and who remained unaware of the implications of their prescriptions for the patient. Treatments, which involved the use of very greasy lotions, posed problems for sufferers and also for their families. They involved hours of work in applying to the skin, were visible and came off on sheets and furniture, and provided only short term relief. This Jobling described as the 'Sysyphus syndrome' (Jobling, 1988, p. 234). In Greek mythology, Sysyphus was condemned by the Gods to roll a huge boulder up a steep mountain. Just before the summit, the rock would roll out of his grasp and down the mountain forcing him to repeat his task again and again.

As stated above, another disease where stigma is a major factor is epilepsy but, unlike psoriasis which is highly visible, the person with epilepsy can often manage the illness so that it remains hidden, and the stigma discreditable. In his research on the experience of epilepsy Scambler (1989) has commented on the historical and cultural specificity of the medical definition of epilepsy, which demonstrates that medical diagnoses are far from fixed categories. However, contemporary medicine classifies epilepsy by type and severity of seizure, a typology that may have little relevance for the person concerned. In interviews with people with epilepsy, Scambler found that much stigma was the result of expectation rather than experience, and that the sense of felt stigma lead to a secrecy that protected against enacted stigma. The biggest source of tension between the participants in the study and the medical profession was the latter's seeming preoccupation with diagnosis and treatment, and a failure to understand the impact of stigma on the lives of people with epilepsy.

This body of work has been criticized by those such as Bury (1991) who argues that much sociological research on chronic illness focused on the problems that people faced, rather than their responses to them. It is also disease specific and therefore reinforces and privileges a biomedical model of disease categorization (Bury, 1997).

However, interpretive perspectives do seek to understand chronic illness through the experiences of people with chronic illnesses themselves. It has moved beyond a simple biomedical categorization of disease to explore the impact that living with it has on the individual and their family. It provided a corrective to the practitioner views that dominated policy and practice in the area (Charmaz, 2000).

Chronic illness as biographical disruption

One of the most important developments in the study of chronic illness came in the 1980s with the work carried out by Bury who argued that much existing sociological research on chronic illness such as that described above, while valuable, focused on the problems that people faced, rather than their responses to them. He proposed the idea of chronic illness as a major disruptive experience in life, and argued that illness, particularly chronic illness is 'the kind of experience where the structures of everyday life and the forms of knowledge which underpin them are disrupted.' (Bury, 1982, p. 169). Biographical disruption is the term used by Bury to describe the assault on one's identity and sense of self worth occasioned by the onset of chronic illness. Disruption occurs in the experience of pain, suffering, and the possibility of death, experiences that have previously been remote, or the plight of others; in the disruption of the normal family and network relationships, such as the physical dependence of a parent on their child; and in the reassessment of plans for the future. All of these issues turn our 'taken for granted' life into a critical situation.

One of the differences between acute and chronic illness is the insidiousness of onset and it is usually some time before the trivial symptoms are considered persistent or severe enough for help seeking behaviour (for the complex nature of help seeking behaviour, see Zola, 1973). For the people with rheumatoid arthritis in Bury's study the involvement of others (both lay and professional) was not until a fairly late stage, although this will differ according to many factors, including the perceived importance of the presenting symptoms. In this and later work, Bury (1991, p. 456) noted that some conditions 'may produce symptoms, which because of their widespread occurrence in milder forms, among the normal population, make legitimation extremely difficult.'

Next is the problem of uncertainty, which is more of an issue in the case of chronic than acute illness. Williams (2003, p. 97, original emphasis) sums this up as '*diagnostic* uncertainty, *symptomatic* uncertainty and *trajectory* uncertainty'. Many studies point to what Robinson (1988) has called the medical merry-go-round of people trying to achieve a diagnosis or some kind of meaning or explanation for what is happening to them, and finding a treatment for the cause of their illness. The success or otherwise of finding a reasonable explanation for the illness, and legitimation (a concept that will be returned to later) can mitigate or compound biographical disruption.

Finally Bury points to attempts at normalizing behaviour, and to the effort involved in maintaining the former everyday world which, because of physical limitations or embarrassment at difficulties encountered, can no longer be 'taken for granted'. However, as he later wrote 'loss of confidence in the body leads to loss of confidence in social interaction.' (Bury, 1991, p. 453). The key themes referred to here of legitimation, uncertainty, and response to chronic illness will be referred to in other chapters of the book.

In subsequent work Bury distinguishes two types of meaning in chronic illness – consequence and significance (Bury, 1988; 1991). Consequence is the effect of the onset of symptoms of long-term illness on all aspects of life, the disruption of a previously 'normal' life. Advice may be taken to deal with symptoms, to manage the altered life, but these often involve a trade off, in terms of the time required to adhere to medical regimes or the effects on other aspects of life. The significance of chronic illness is the imagery conjured up by the condition, influenced by social and cultural norms, by the person concerned and by others. It is this that affects the sense of self, and the reaction of others to the condition. The impact of this significance on the person and on his/her social relationships will often be negative but this is not inevitable. Significance is not static and may change, for example over the life course when older people, and those around them, may interpret certain symptoms as a normal part of ageing.

While this work has been important in developing a socio-logical analysis of chronic illness, in particular one that gives prominence and legitimacy to the lay voice, it has not been uncritically accepted, and Williams (2003) provides a useful summary of critiques of biographically informed perspectives, including the concept of biographical disruption. Firstly, the notion of an impaired body causing biographical disruption renders medical sociology complicit in a medicalized approach to disability, one that has more in common with a personal tragedy stance than a view of disability as social oppression. Second, postmodernists criticize the fixed categories of mod-ernist thinking and look to a more relative, or contingent rela-tionship than either a biomedical or structural model propose. However, there are, suggests Williams, more useful observa-tions to be made about biographical disruption that move the concept forward. The first concerns that fact that the whole notion of disruption assumes a previous undisrupted state, which makes it a somewhat adult-centric model. For those who are born with chronic conditions, or develop them in early childhood there is often no shift from a normal to a diseased state, the condition or disease is integral to a person's 'bio-graphically embodied sense of self' (Williams, 2003, p. 103). The second issue draws upon work carried out on lay defini-tion of illness, such as those of Blaxter and Patterson (1982) and Cornwell (1984) who differentiate between 'normal' and 'serious', or 'normal' and 'real' illness. 'Normal' illness is to be expected and endured. Much of this research was conducted with people who experience much adversity in life of which illness or disabling conditions are just one aspect, one crisis among many. Similarly and more recently, Fairclough et al. (2004, p. 245) in their narrative research on the stroke recov-ery experience in the United States of America argue that 'a sudden illness, such as stroke, does not always serve as a dis-ruptive event, but instead melds into an enduring chronic ill-ness narrative, part-and-parcel of biography.'

What these examples point to is what Kelly and Field (1998) argue is increasing diversity in the experience of chronic ill-ness afforded by changes in society. Without being absolut-ist they point to the shift from modernity to post-modernity, from a more stable economic and class base to a society that is more fragmented and diverse, for example witness the range of ethnic groups currently inhabiting most of the Western world, and the complexity of modern family structure. Kelly and Field point to the notion of stigma and spoiled identity (discussed above) in which appearance that was different or disfigured was always negatively viewed by oneself and others. Inspired by the disability movement (see below), they argue that there is now not only a celebration of difference, but an attack on the ideological assumption of normality. However, post-modernism is nothing if it is not Janus headed (pointing in both directions at the same time) and it could be argued that the increasing drive for physical perfection encouraged by the media and cosmetic surgery industry has made physical differences less acceptable, and something to be corrected. An example here is the growth in facial surgery on those people with Down's Syndrome (Aylott, 1999).

Illness narratives

While Bury argued that biographical disruption was caused by the experience of chronic illness, other sociological litera-ture has shown how narratives are used by people to explain illness within the context of their biography, in other words disruption precedes and is a factor in the development of ill health. Gareth Williams (1989) outlines two aspects of 'narra-tive' when used as a sociological concept. In its routine form it refers to the observations and comment on the everyday events of life, the order given to mundane events. When the mun-dane is thrown into disarray or confusion, what he calls 'nar-rative reconstruction' (p. 268) is an attempt by people to make sense of what is happening to them. 'Narrative reconstruction therefore represents the workings of the discursive conscious-ness' (p. 270). Williams illustrates this in his research on the experience of arthritis, where the participants use narrative to make sense of the illness in terms of their past biography and to explain its genesis. For example Bill, one of the respondents in Williams' study, viewed the genesis of his illness as extrane-ous, from the chemicals he worked with and the long hours in the workplace whereas Gill, another respondent, internalized it and explained her arthritis as being related to stressful events and suppression of herself in favour of husband and children.

Hydén (1997, p. 49) states that 'one of our most powerful forms for expressing suffering and experiences related to suffering is the narrative. Patients' narratives give voice to suffering in away that lies outside the domain of the biomedical voice.' Hydén categorized illness narratives as a typology based on 'the *formal* aspects of illness narratives; namely, the relationship between narrator, narrative and illness' (Hydén, 1997, p. 54, original emphasis). These, he suggests, may interrelate to give rise to at least three types of illness narrative, illness *as* narrative, narrative *about* illness, and narrative *as* illness. In the first type illness is articulated and expressed through narrative. The illness, the narrator and the narrative may be combined in the same person. This encompasses the person's story regarding the occurrence of the illness, and the way in which it is accommodated into the totality of that person's life. Thus it is possible to integrate symptoms and consequences of illness into a new being. The second type, narrative about illness is primarily about the illness, rather than the person, and constructs and conveys knowledge and ideas about illness. Health professionals use narratives about illness to gain information on the patient's illness, to reach a diagnosis and to formulate acceptable treatment regimes. Hydén's third type, narrative as illness, reflects the instances when the inability to narrate or to articulate is a crucial aspect of illness, as in the case of brain injury. The consequence of narrative for the process and product of research is explored further in Chapter 3.

The sociology of disability and the social model of disability

Chronic illness is a major cause of disability in western societies, and increasingly so in developing societies. As such disability theory and the sociology of disability can be useful in making sense of the explosion of chronic illness in society. Traditionally disability has been seen as a medical problem, caused by some physical or mental impairment, and many disabled people were segregated in residential institutions of one sort or another. Disability was seen as the resulting restrictions in function and activity of the impairment, a view evident in the World Health Organization definitions published as the International Classification of Impairments, Disabilities and Handicaps (WHO, 1980). Impairment referred to the abnormality of the structure of the body (epilepsy, paraplegia), disability referred to the restriction in the ability to carry out tasks and functions, and handicap was the social disadvantage associated with either impairment or disability (Bury, 1997). This definition has now been updated and is known as the ICF – or International Classification of Functioning, Disability and Health (WHO, 2001) This definition, which focuses on body function and activity, as well as on environment factors has been described as a 'radical shift' in thinking about disability and health (WHO, 2002, p. 3). This discussion, of course, does beg the question of why such definitions and frameworks are important and how they might be of relevance to practice. The WHO argues that the ICF framework is:

> ...the conceptual basis for the definition, measurement and policy formulations for health and disability. It is a universal classification of disability *and* health for use in health and health-related sectors. (WHO, 2002, p. 2)

In other words, such frameworks provide a blueprint for the ways in which disabled people are perceived within health, as well as within society more generally. Within this individualized model, disability is viewed as a personal tragedy for the individual and the goal of policy is to adapt the individual by rehabilitation and physical and financial aid to the environment of the non-disabled. By focusing on the impairment, disability becomes a medically defined problem, and if cure is not possible, it is up to the disabled individual to adjust as far as possible to their environment in order to overcome their disadvantage. The needs of the disabled person are defined by the medical profession, which also controls the means of meeting them. Along with a welfarist model that responds to disability with awards of services and benefits, this disempowers the individual who is seen as a victim in need of professional help, and who is viewed in terms of his/her limitations. This attitude is not confined to health services, but also operates in education and employment, where opportunities for people with disabilities are limited by assumptions that are made about what disabled people can (or more likely cannot) do.

The social model, on the other hand, regards disability not as a personal issue but a societal one. It rejects any automatic link between impairment and disability. Disabled people are not handicapped by their impairment, but by the structures of society that prevent them from participating fully in social, political and economic life. They are disadvantaged by discrimination and exclusion from mainstream society. Disability thus becomes redefined as a form of social oppression (Thomas, 2004). The social model recognizes the need for self determination and autonomy in making decisions about how to live one's life, not merely being *given* a choice in mundane issues – such as which television channel to watch! In short, disability theory defines disability as a social issue, rather than as a medical one; the justification for this being that whilst disabled people may be or become ill (just as a non-disabled person might) the disabled person is not ill *because* they are disabled.

Of course, whilst the social model of disability has helped shift attention away from medicine and the individual towards locating disability within the social structures of society, some sociologists have been critical of this model arguing that it does little to help explain the lived experiences of those with long-term conditions. These critiques are examined next.

The sociology of the body

As some people who have been disabled as a result of living with chronic illness have argued, disability theory is useful in that it has persuaded some health and social care professionals to adopt a more empowering approach within their work. However, disability theory does not really help to make sense of the limitations posed when living with disorientation, low mood, pain, discomfort or poor mobility. Some theorists, such as Pinder (1995) have argued that disability theory, and the social model in particular, has taken a disembodied approach to disability. Indeed, Williams and Busby (2000) suggest that the social model has ignored bodily change and decay.

Traditionally, sociology sought to differentiate itself from the more positivistic natural sciences by focusing on society and by rejecting essentialist perspectives which define phenomena as 'natural' or fixed. Essentialism – which could be described as a form of biological determinism – views phenomena (such as race or sex) as unchanging, rather than as something which is socially and culturally constructed. As such, some sociologists have argued that this has led to the neglect of the body within sociology, leaving an analytical gap at the core of sociological theory (Turner, 1984; 1995). The sociology of the body, which began to develop in the 1990s, encompasses work which seeks to bring the body 'back in' (Frank, 1990) to sociological inquiry and it has enormous relevance for a sociology of long-term conditions.

Sociologists tend to approach the study of the body in one of two different ways. Some sociologists are interested in the body as 'lived experience'. It is an approach which often draws on interpretivist and narrative methods. The majority of studies on long-term conditions have adopted such an approach in that they are concerned with exploring 'what it is like' to live with – or with someone who has – a particular condition. Examples of these include Miklaucich's (1998) study of women living with angina major, Harman and Clare's (2006) study of people with early-stage dementia and Prasomsuk et al.'s (2007) study of mothers who care for children living with Thalassaemia. Other sociologists are interested in the construction of the body and in the way that the body is a representation of culture. Foucault (1977), for example, has described the body as the direct locus of control for society, subject to external forces which 'mark it', 'train it' and 'force it to carry out tasks' (1977, p. 25). Many studies draw on both interpretivist and constructionist approaches to the body.

One condition which has received considerable attention within the sociology of the body is that of chronic pain, and this has had important consequences for nursing practice. Sociologists, for example, have highlighted the way in which pain is a subjective and individual experience, demonstrating the importance of individualized nursing practice (Clarke and Iphofen, 2005). In particular, studies have shown that patients living with chronic pain are often not believed. In a study of women living with fibromyalgia (Råheim and Håland, 2006), participants report feelings of powerlessness and despair. One respondent, Maren, describes the 'constant hell of pain': 'It takes ages to get out of bed and into the bathroom. It is like moving mountains. I'm so extremely stiff, and the pain is just unbearable. It's just pain and pain!' (p. 747). In the light of findings such as these some authors have considered the importance for sufferers of legitimation of their pain, both as a vindication of themselves, and to gain access or to improve relations within the health care system. Werner and Malterud (2003), for example, report on the work that women with medically unexplained pain do in order to be taken seriously by doctors. The women in their study invested much time and effort in trying to project the image of a credible patient, assessing the amount of assertiveness to display or how to dress in what they describe as a bodily and engendered balance (Werner and Malterud, 2003) (see Chapter 12 for a further discussion of pain).

The subject of sexuality and chronic illness has also received attention by sociologists. For many people living with a long-term condition, sexuality is impaired or transformed by the experience of pain and impairment, or due to the pharmacological effects of prescription medication. Living with a long-term condition can have far-reaching consequences for everyday life a well as for self-identity. For example, in a study of women living with chronic vulvar pain – which limits the capacity to engage in penetrative vaginal intercourse – women described themselves as inadequate and genderless (Kaler, 2006). Norma, one participant in this study stated: '[I feel like] a freak. I feel like I'm not a woman. That part of what a woman is has been denied to me. I want to have sexual intercourse and have babies and knowing that it might be impossible for me makes me very depressed' (Kaler, 2006, p. 60). Difficulties with sexuality have also been expressed by people with diabetes and arthritis. Of course, people living with a long-term condition do not always encounter difficulties with sexual activity or expression. For example, in a study of women with lupus, Karlen (2002) notes that, despite a range of disabling symptoms, many women were able to actually enhance their sexual function and enjoyment. However, Karlen argues that: 'Patients too rarely bring up these subjects, and health professionals too rarely ask' thus highlighting the need for better communication between practitioners and their clients (p. 207).

Summary

This chapter has taken a historical approach in order to provide an overview of some of the more influential work in the sociology of chronic illness. It has demonstrated how changing sociological perspectives of chronic illness have reflected the changing nature of sociological inquiry more generally. The early work of sociologists in studying specific diseases, made visible for the first time the experience of people whose suffering had previously been invisible. The work of interactionists analyzed the meaning of experience for individuals, thus providing a corrective to the previously dominant medical practitioner view of illness. Hydén (1997) points to the way that the body of knowledge that constitutes a sociological analysis of chronic illness has highlighted the individual's experience, perspective and interpretation. The biomedical model with its focus on organs, pathological changes and measurable deviations from some medically defined norm was characterised by scepticism of accounts by patients.

Early sociological studies also took as their starting point biomedically defined and conceptualised illness. The separation of illness from disease and the later shift to the suffering caused by illness, opened the way for patient narratives to be explored as credible and crucial sources of knowledge. Although there are those who argue that this separation created a false distinction, the usefulness of the work created cannot be overstated. Later, structuralist sociologists looked to the institutions of society, such as the welfare or education systems, to explain the disadvantage and discrimination experienced by those who were incapacitated by their chronic illness. More recent post-modernist work has recognized the diversity and fluidity of human experience and moved away from the generalities and universalizing tendency of some early work. The inter-relationship between different social factors, such as age, gender, and ethnicity, and the experience of chronic illness has been acknowledged. Also acknowledged is the dynamism of the experience of individuals, for example over the life course.

The sociology of chronic illness, then, has over the years provided a fascinating insight into the world of those who experience it. It has considered individual disease states, but has also taken a more generalized approach, one which does not rely on medical diagnoses. For nurses a sociological perspective is a vital addition to the biomedical perspectives that continue to dominate the knowledge base of the profession.

References

Armstrong D., 'Chronic illness: epidemiological or social explosion', *Chronic Illness*, 1: 1 (2005) 26–27.

Aylott J., 'Should children with Down's syndrome have cosmetic surgery?', *British Journal of Nursing*, 8: 1 (1999) 33–38.

Blaxter M. and E. Patterson, *Mothers and Daughters: a Three Generational Study of Health Attitudes and Behaviour* (London: Heinemann, 1982).

Bury M., 'Chronic illness as biographical disruption', *Sociology of Health & Illness*, 4: 2(1982) 167–182.

Bury M., 'Meanings at risk: the experience of arthritis', in R. Anderson and M. Bury (eds), *Living with Chronic Illness: The Experience of Patients and their Families* (London: Unwin Hyman, 1988).

Bury M., 'The sociology of chronic illness', *Sociology of Health & Illness*, 13: 4 (1991) 263–285.

Bury M., *Health and Illness in a Changing Society* (London: Routledge, 1997).

Chapple A., S. Ziebland and A. McPherson, 'Stigma, shame and blame experienced by patients with lung cancer: qualitative study', *British Medical Journal*, 328: 7454 (2004) 1470–1473.

Charmaz K., 'Experiencing chronic illness', in G.L. Albrecht, R. Fitzpatrick, S.C. Scrimshaw (eds), *The Handbook of Social Studies in Health and Medicine* (London: Sage, 2000).

Clarke K.A., and R. Iphofen, 'Believing the patient with chronic pain: a review of the literature', *British Journal of Nursing*, 14: 9 (2005) 490–493.

Cornwell J., *Hard Earned Lives* (London: Tavistock, 1984).

Corrigan P.W., and F.E. Miller, 'Shame, blame and contamination: A review of the impact of mental illness stigma on family members', *Journal of Mental Health*, 13: 6 (2004) 537–548.

Fairclough C.A., C. Boylstein, M. Rittman, M.E. Young and J. Gubrium, 'Sudden illness and biographical flow in narratives of stroke recovery', *Sociology of Health and Illness*, 26 (2004) 242–261.

Foucault M., *Discipline and Punish, the Birth of the Prison* (Harmondsworth: Penguin, 1977).

Frank A.W., 'Bringing bodies back in: a decade review', *Theory, Culture and Society*, 7 (1990) 131–162.

Fraser S., and C. Treloar, '"Spoiled identity" in hepatitis C infection: The binary logic of despair', *Critical Public Health*, 16: 2 (2006) 99–110.

Gerhardt U., 'Parsons, role theory, and health interaction', in G. Scambler (ed.), *Sociological Theory and Medical Sociology* (London: Routledge, 1987).

Goffman E., *Stigma: Notes on the Management of a Spoiled Identity* (London: Penguin Books, 1963).

Harman G., and L. Clare, 'Illness representations and lived experience in early-stage dementia', *Qualitative Health Research*, 16: 4 (2006) 484–502.

Hydén L.C., 'Illness and narrative', *Sociology of Health and Illness*, 19: 1 (1997) 48–69.

Jobling R., 'The experience of Psoriasis under treatment', in R. Anderson and M. Bury (eds), *Living with Chronic Illness: The Experience of Patients and their Families* (London: Unwin Hyman, 1988) 225–244.

Kaler A., 'Unreal women: sex, gender, identity and the lived experience of vulvar pain', *Feminist Review*, 82 (2006) 50–75.

Karlen A., 'Positive sexual effects of chronic illness: case studies of women living with lupus (SLE)', *Sexuality and Disability*, 20: 3 (2002) 191–208.

Macrae H., 'Managing courtesy stigma: the case of Alzheimer's disease', *Sociology of Health & Illness*, 21: 1 (1999) 54–70.

May C., 'Chronic illness and intractability: professional-patient interactions in primary care', *Chronic Illness*, 1: 1 (2005) 15–20.

Miklaucich M., 'Limitations on life: women's lived experiences of angina', *Journal of Advanced Nursing*, 28: 6 (1998) 1207–1215.

Oliver M., *Social Work with Disabled People* (Basingstoke: Macmillan, 1983).

Parsons T., *The Social System* (London: Routledge and Kegan Paul, 1951).

Pinder R., 'Bringing back the body without the blame? The experience of ill and disabled people at work', *Sociology of Health and Illness*, 17: 5 (1995) 605–631.

Prasomsuk S., A. Jetsrisuparp, T. Ratanasiri and A. Ratanasiri, 'Lived experiences of mothers caring for children with Thalassemia Major In Thailand', *Journal for Specialists in Pediatric Nursing,* 12: 1 (2007) 13–23.

Råheim M., and W. Håland, 'Lived experience of chronic pain and fibromyalgia: women's stories from daily life', *Qualitative Health Research,* 16: 6 (2006) 741–761.

Robinson I., *Multiple Sclerosis* (London: Routledge, 1988).

Roth J.A., *Timetables: Structuring the Passage of Time in Hospital Treatment and Other Careers* (Indianapolis: Bobbs Merrill, 1963).

Scambler G., *Epilepsy* (London: Tavistock/Routledge, 1989).

Scambler G., 'Sociology, social structure and health-related stigma', *Psychology, Health and Medicine,* 11: 3 (2006) 288–295.

Shilling C., 'Culture, the "sick role" and the consumption of health', *British Journal of Sociology,* 53: 4 (2002) 621–638.

Sontag S., *Illness and Metaphor* (London: Allen Lane, 1979).

Thomas C., 'Disability and impairment', in J. Swain, S. French, C. Barnes, and C. Thomas (eds), *Disabling Barriers: Enabling Environments* 2nd edn (London: Sage, 2004).

Turner B.S., *The Body and Society: Explorations in Social Theory* (Oxford: Basil Blackwell, 1984).

Turner B.S., *Medical Power, Social Knowledge* 2nd edn (London: Sage, 1995).

Van Brakel W., 'Measuring health-related stigma – a literature review', *Psychology, Health and Medicine,* 11: 3 (2006) 307–334.

Werner A., and K. Malterud, 'It is hard behaving as a credible patient: encounters between women with chronic pain and their doctors', *Social Science and Medicine,* 57: 8 (2003) 1409–1419.

Williams G., 'The genesis of chronic illness: narrative re-construction', in P. Brown (ed.), *Perspectives in Medical Sociology* (Belmont, California: Wadsworth, 1989).

Williams I., and H. Busby, 'The politics of disabled bodies', in S.J. Williams, J. Gabe and M. Calnan (eds), *Health, Medicine and Society* (London: Routledge, 2000).

Williams S.J., *Medicine and the Body* (London: Sage, 2003).

Williams S.J., 'Parsons revisited: from the sick role to...?', *Health: An Interdisciplinary Journal for the Social Study of Health, Illness & Medicine,* 9: 2 (2005) 123–144.

Wilson K., and K. Luker, 'At home in hospital? Interaction and stigma in people affected by cancer', *Social Science and Medicine,* 62 (2006) 1616–1627.

World Health Organization (WHO), *International Classification of Impairments, Disabilities and Handicaps: a Manual of*

Classification Relating to the Consequences of Disease (Geneva: WHO, 1980).

World Health Organization (WHO), *Resolution of the World Health Assembly*. Fifty-fourth World Health Assembly (Geneva: WHO, 2001) http://www3.who.int/icf/whares/wha-en.pdf (last accessed 5 November 2007).

World Health Organization (WHO), *Towards a Common Language for Functioning, Disability and Health: ICF* (Geneva: WHO, 2002) http://www3.who.int/icf/beginners/bg.pdf (last accessed 5 November 2007).

Zola I.K., 'Pathways to the doctor: from person to patient', *Social Science and Medicine*, 7 (1973) 677–689.

2 Long term conditions, policy and practice

Alistair Hewison and David Cox

Introduction

> Chronic illness constitutes a major health policy issue: How can we deal with the manifestation and effects of this presently incurable and prevalent form of illness? ...the prevalence of chronic illness necessitates profound changes in our health care system and our society itself.
>
> *(Strauss and Corbin, 1988, p. xi)*

These words written in 1988 have proved to be somewhat prophetic. As Ham (2005a) observes, people are now living longer lives. However the number of years of healthy life has not increased at the same rate as overall life expectancy. This means that people are living more years in poor health or with a limiting long term illness. Conditions like arthritis, diabetes and depression affect a large number of people and are more common in older than younger age groups. People with more than one condition are at greater risk of becoming heavy users of health services and consuming a disproportionate share of healthcare resources (Ham, 2005a). In the United Kingdom, 17.5 million people report having a long term condition (Department of Health (DH), 2005d, see introduction for a discussion of definitions). This presents a significant challenge because our health care system, being in common with most of the Western Democracies, is designed primarily for treating acute and episodic illness (Canadian Health Services Research Foundation, 2005). Acute hospital care can stabilize patients; however it makes little contribution to the on-going well being of the patient. Moreover, it can actually expose them to the risks of infection and institutionalization. This means we need to move away from managing care on the basis of discrete periods of treatment in hospital when people become seriously ill, towards the provision of continuous high quality care delivered by teams combining specialist expertise and generalist capabilities. It is also important to involve patients and their families more directly in the provision of care (Ham, 2005a). How is this challenge being met in the United Kingdom? In order to answer this question a number of areas need to be considered. First, a brief discussion of the policy process will be presented to provide some context; this is followed by a summary of the scale of the problem and a discussion of the policy response; finally the implications for nursing will be examined.

The policy process

Hennessy (2000) contends that the shape of nursing is determined by health policy. Similarly Hart (2004) maintains that if we are to understand nursing and its practice we have to be prepared to develop a perspective on politics and power. To a large extent policies are the outcome of the interplay of politics and power. Consequently, some appreciation of how the policy process works is necessary if nurses are to deliver the care required by patients with long term conditions, or indeed any other group of patients. However, presenting a straightforward definition of the term is difficult because it has a number of elements. Ham and Hill (1993) suggest that policy involves a course of action or a web of decisions rather than one decision. This series of decisions can take place over a period of time and the nature of the policy itself can change during the conduct of the process. So health policy is not simply what is laid out in national strategy documents; it is also about how those strategies are put into practice on the ground by health care professionals, patients and the wider community who are the object of the policy change (Green and Thorogood, 1998). In other words, 'the authoritative statements of intent about action which relate to the maintenance of good health in individuals and populations; the cure of disease and illness; and the care of the vulnerable and the frail' (Allsop, 1995, p. 4) are often only the starting point. These statements can be generated from a number of sources (see below) and in being implemented, the resultant policies may be, and indeed often are, changed by the interpretations, actions or inertia of the range of people working in health and social care. Also these distortions can reflect the relative power of the individuals or groups involved (Allsop, 1995).

This indicates that policy can be viewed and considered on a number of different levels. Hudson and Lowe (2004) suggest a three-way classification for these purposes:

The **macro-level** (macro being derived from the Greek word *macros* meaning long, extensive) encompassing the broad parameters that shape policy: for example globalization, the global market place.

The **meso-level** concerns the practice of the policy making process itself and the institutions engaged in designing and seeing policy through to its delivery. They argue that it is crucially embedded in what they identify as policy networks. These are made up of a range of organizations and agencies that initiate filter and shape policy outcomes. For example the Department of Health, as part of the government sets the overall policy direction; however, it is influenced by other 'inputs'. Research centres and Think Tanks, such as the King's Fund in London, produce data and comment, which affect government thinking in this area for example, Wanless et al., 2007. Also the National Health Service (NHS) Confederation, which represents many NHS Trusts, produces comment on behalf of Trusts intended to affect policy decisions. Similarly professional organizations, including the Royal College of Nursing, seek to lobby government on nursing and health issues. The **micro-level** focuses down onto two themes, engagement between consumers and agencies, and between individuals. This directs attention to where policy is enacted at the point of care delivery: first in the experience of patients as receivers of services, second in the actions of practitioners and clients as shapers of policy as it is implemented.

This provides a schema for thinking about the complicated business of policy. It is not just about the actions of government. It is also about how diverse interest groups, research evidence, the influence of the media and the actions of individuals all come together to shape the content and outcome of policy. As noted above, nursing as a discipline can also play a significant part in this process. Nurses, midwives and health visitors make up the largest number of health professionals and the biggest staff group in the NHS and consequently the nature of nursing work and the profession of nursing itself are fully intertwined with health and social policy development (Masterson, 2002). Walt (1994) argues that for most people policy is concerned with content, such as the best method for financing health services or improving health care delivery, whilst for others it is about process and power. It is a very complex area and as Masterson (1994) observes it seems everyone who writes about social policy offers a definition, and discussions concerning the exact nature of anything can often become pedantic and tedious. The approach taken here is to present a relatively simple explanation of the policy process (see below) and direct attention to the reference list as a source of suggestions for further reading which can be accessed for more detail. The intention is to provide a context for the discussion of policy in the area of long term conditions in the United Kingdom, rather than to engage in an in-depth analysis of the policy process itself.

One way of thinking about the policy process is to consider how an issue gets on to the 'agenda' and leads to action. Ham (2004) argues that in order for a policy issue to lead to action it has to meet certain requirements. It must:

- Attract attention
- Claim legitimacy
- Invoke action. (Ham, 2004 [after Solesbury, 1976])

In relation to the policy area of long term conditions, the fact that more people are living longer and experiencing poorer health has 'attracted attention' because it presents a challenge to health services. It 'claims legitimacy' because it is accepted by the government that resources and policy should be directed towards addressing this issue. Finally it is 'invoking action' in that measures are being put in place to provide new models of care and intervention for this client group. This perspective on the policy process can also be regarded as the opening of a 'policy window' (Brehaut and Juzwishin, 2005). A policy window opens when three streams come together. These streams are problems, proposals, and politics. In sum, policy decisions are made when a problem is recognized, policy solutions are available, and the political conditions are right (Brehaut and Juzwishin, 2005; Kingdon, 1984). In the case of health care, ideology, expediency and public preferences compete with scientific evidence for the ears of ministers (Davies et al., 1999). Issues can be identified as requiring action because they are felt to be important by the government, the focus of this chapter for example – long term conditions. High profile media coverage can create a 'crisis' or push an issue to the top of the policy agenda. In the case of long term conditions the 'tipping point' has been the impact on acute hospital services (Hudson, 2005). The number of people with long term conditions receiving care in acute hospitals has jeopardized the highly prized achievement of political targets in the areas of waiting times and access (Hudson, 2005). There are many 'voices', which input to the policy process and this can be regarded as a good thing. 6 (2002) contends that in a democratic polity, policy making should reflect a whole range of types of information that are counted as evidence. Inevitably though this means the making of policy is 'messy' and confusing. It can appear to (and sometimes does) lack direction, and policies can work counter to each other. For example in another area of policy the *Choosing Health* (DH, 2005b) approach to encouraging people to take more responsibility for a healthy lifestyle could be regarded as having limited potential for success unless other areas of policy such as transport and the environment are addressed. It is difficult for people to choose exercise if cycle lanes or playing fields are not available. Similarly the themes of regulation and self-management, which have characterized the government's approach to policy overall, are inherently contradictory (Crinson, 2005). NHS Trusts are encouraged to become self-managing organizations in the form of Foundation Trusts and yet are subjected to an increasing amount of regulation and inspection (Walshe, 2002). This has led some commentators to conclude that there is no overarching strategy discernible among the hotch-potch of change occurring, and little continuity for those attempting to implement the government's agenda (Greener, 2004). Consequently policy is not a rational, objective, neutral activity devoid of values or the play of power. Individuals and groups in health care organizations have multiple and conflicting objectives and interests and their desire to defend these is an important determinant of policy outcomes (Hunter, 2003). Thus, the interface between policy and practice may be characterized by ambiguity of intent and unpredictability of response, making it both complex and problematic (Bergen and While, 2005). These factors need to be taken into account when considering the introduction of a policy framework for the management of long term conditions, as they constitute the context in which the policy has been developed and applied.

The policy problem

Given that 17.5 million people in the United Kingdom report having a long term condition (DH, 2005d) it is important to demonstrate what this means in practical terms and why it has attracted attention, claimed legitimacy and invoked action as a major policy concern. The presentation of a range of figures is helpful in explaining some of the reasons this issue has risen to the top of the policy agenda. Wilson et al. (2005) draw on an analysis of the British Household Panel Survey (2001) and the General Household Survey (2001) to identify the scale of the problem:

- Six in ten adults in the United Kingdom report some form of chronic health problem
- People with chronic health problems account for 80 per cent of General Practitioner (GP) consultations
- Use of health care services increases in line with the number of conditions reported. The 15 per cent of the people with three or more chronic conditions account for 30 per cent of in-patient days
- People with long term conditions are twice as likely to be intensive users of services than those without

Consequently two thirds of emergency hospital admissions in Britain involve people with long term conditions (Singh, 2005), the cost of health care associated with chronic disease accounts for a growing proportion of health expenditure

(Hutt and Rosen, 2005) and most importantly chronic diseases are now the main cause of death and disability worldwide (Groves and Wagner, 2005).

In the United Kingdom, this means that 10 per cent of patients with long term conditions account for 55 per cent of in-patient days (Hudson, 2005). Another way of thinking about this is that arguably at any one time more than half the patients in hospital would be better cared for elsewhere. This indicates that the needs of these patients are not being met in the acute setting and that the lack of suitable alternative provision is preventing the system from doing what it was set up to achieve (Hudson, 2005).

There is also a major economic concern here. For patients with more than one condition, costs are six times higher than those with only one, and 78 per cent of all healthcare spend relates to people with long term conditions (DH, 2004a). This, combined with the estimate that by 2030 the incidence of long term disease in those who are over the age of 65 years will more than double (DH, 2004a), serves to demonstrate why the organization of care for people with long term conditions has become a pressing policy concern.

If the system is struggling to cope with patients with complex long term conditions it cannot meet the needs of other patients requiring elective surgery and acute care. Also the current organization of services, based on a model of providing people requiring acute time limited interventions with treatment and care, now has a fundamental design fault. It is not 'fit for purpose' in that it cannot meet the needs of the majority of its users, those with long term conditions. Also the continuing escalation in health care costs as the number of patients in this category increases represents another significant challenge. The Department of Health has been set a target to achieve efficiency savings of 2.7 per cent per year over the period 2005/06 to 2007/08. The intention is that these savings will be achieved through a mixture of cost efficiency and quality improvements and include savings made in the NHS, Adult Social Care, and the management of the Department of Health itself (DH, 2004b). Delivering cost savings in the face of increasing demands on the health care budget constitutes a major problem for policy makers.

The policy response

This is a challenge in most of the Western Democracies. Many countries, including the United States, Australia, Canada and the United Kingdom, have focused on the management of patients with long term conditions, targeting in particular those who use health services a lot (Hutt and Rosen, 2005). The 'Global nature' of this policy issue has resulted in some sharing of information and the adoption of similar responses across nations. The English strategy has been influenced by the United States and can be thought of as a hybrid 'Anglo–US' model (Hudson, 2005), and the similarities to the Kaiser Permanente structure (see below) indicate how policy responses can be transferred across national boundaries. This is not unusual in policy creation as West and Scott (2000), drawing on the work of Kingdon (1984), observe: 'Solutions to problems are not generally designed anew. Ideas and policies swim around, mutate, metamorphose, reproduce and die in the cultural equivalent of a "primeval soup". Policy makers can often find in this pool of ideas a solution that is more or less applicable to any situation' (West and Scott, 2000, p. 819).

In this case the Department of Health has looked to other nations for a solution to the UK situation through a process of policy transfer (Hulme, 2005). This is based on an assumption that targeting intensive packages of care at these high-risk individuals can reduce hospital admissions. The specific targets for providers of health care in the United Kingdom are:

- Reduce in-patient bed days by 5 per cent by March 2008
- Offer a personalized care plan for vulnerable people most at risk (DH, 2005c)

In order to do this those working in health care are required to design and redesign services using the NHS and Social Care Long Term Conditions Model. This is based on the Kaiser Permanente system and includes an adaptation of the 'pyramid of care'. This pyramid of care 'segments' the population of patients with long term conditions into three levels, which reflect their degree of need (see Figure 2.1).

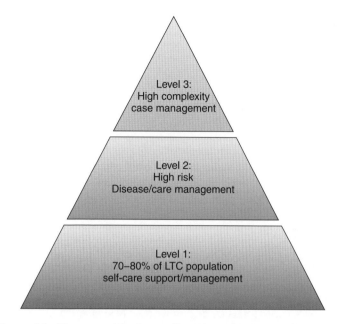

Figure 2.1 The pyramid of care (based on the Kaiser Permanente Model) (DH, 2005d, p. 10)

© Crown copyright, 2005. Crown copyright material is reproduced with the permission of the Controller of HMSO and the Queen's printer for Scotland

A combination of approaches has been applied to achieve help facilitate this and the main elements are outlined below:

Kaiser Permanente

Kaiser Permanente is a long established, not-for-profit health maintenance organization. It was originally set up to offer prepaid medical care to workers in the construction and shipyard industries in the United States, and opened to the public in 1945. In some ways it is similar to the NHS because it functions as an integrated financing and delivery system, however it has been suggested that its results are better (Ham, 2005b). Kaiser integrates prevention, treatment and care. This is most evident in relation to people with chronic diseases such as diabetes and heart failure. They receive structured care from multidisciplinary teams located in the community. Central to the Kaiser system is the 'pyramid of care' (see Figure 2.1) and its philosophy is that unplanned hospital admissions are a sign of failure (Ham, 2005b). The care and intervention required at the different levels of the pyramid are summarized below:

Level 3: Case management – requires the identification of the very high intensity users of unplanned secondary care. Care for these patients is to be managed using a Community Matron or other professional using a case management approach, to anticipate, co-ordinate and join up health and social care.

Level 2: Disease-specific care management – This involves providing people who have a complex single need or multiple conditions with responsive, specialist services using multidisciplinary teams and disease-specific protocols and pathways, such as National Service Frameworks (NSFs) and Quality and Outcomes Framework.

Level 1: Supported self-care – collaboratively helping individuals and their carers to develop the knowledge, skills and confidence to care for themselves and their condition effectively (DH, 2005d; 2005c). This also builds on an earlier Expert Patient initiative (DH, 2001) whereby drawing on patients' knowledge of their own illness is central to care provision.

This is to be achieved through multi-professional teams working together using integrated patient pathways to ensure improved delivery of health and social care, as part of a systematic approach. The basis for this new way of working is illustrated in the NHS and Social Care Long Term Conditions Model.

The NHS and social care long term conditions model

This Model draws on local and international experiences and innovations, to improve the health and quality of life of those with long term conditions. It incorporates elements from Kaiser Permanente, the 'chronic care model' and Evercare, all developed in the United States (DH, 2004a). The purpose of the Model is to improve the health and quality of life of those with long term conditions by providing a mechanism for personalized, yet systematic on-going support, based on what works best for people in NHS and social care systems (DH, 2005d) (see Figure 2.2).

However it is recognized that it will take time before the effects of this are felt. Work is in hand to develop incentives for the whole patient journey, not only the hospital element, and to improve incentives to integrate social care provision into the patient experience (DH, 2004b).

In England, Primary Care Trusts (PCTs) are responsible for the local implementation of health policy and have a budget for meeting the primary and secondary care needs of their residents (between 200,000 and 1 million people). Similar responsibilities fall to the Local Health Boards in Scotland, Wales and Northern Ireland. The PCTs have to develop a

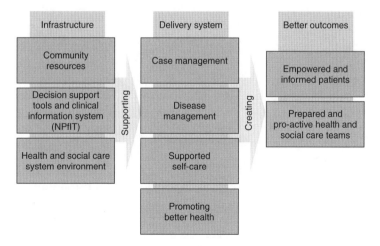

Figure 2.2 The NHS and social care long term conditions model (DH, 2005d, p. 9)

© Crown copyright, 2005. Crown copyright material is reproduced with the permission of the Controller of HMSO and the Queen's printer for Scotland

strategy that will ensure the needs of their patients and service users are met, while as far as possible avoiding unnecessary and costly hospital admissions. Once a patient is seen in the accident and emergency department or admitted to hospital the PCT must pay for the treatment received, even if it is inappropriate or leads to adverse consequences such as hospital borne infections, loss of confidence and mobility or a delayed discharge while social care support is re-organized. In many cases an emergency admission is triggered by a crisis such as a severe asthma attack, breathlessness, a collapse, a fall or a breakdown in social care arrangements. This creates an incentive for the PCTs to work with GPs, case managers, Community Matrons and district nurses to try and anticipate problems and provide better support in the community. An emergency admission to hospital to stabilize a crisis, or repeated admissions to hospital, are symptoms of an inadequate set of monitoring and support arrangements within the primary care and community setting. Improving the care of people with chronic and long term conditions in the community is good health care practice and also makes financial sense. PCTs across the country, in collaboration with local authorities, are now investing in ensuring that people with long term conditions and complex needs are identified. They are also training and developing teams of staff who can respond to crises directly in the patient's home – or better still – provide active case management in partnership with the patient/service user and avoid a crisis in the first place (South Birmingham PCT, 2006).

National service framework (NSF)

However these examples of policy transfer are only part of the policy response. The Department of Health has also produced a NSF for Long Term Conditions. So as well as developing a model for the care and management of patients with long term conditions, the Department has also collated a range of evidence on which to base quality requirements for people with long term neurological conditions (DH, 2005c). Although the NSF focuses on people with neurological conditions, much of the guidance it offers can apply to anyone living with a long term condition and the expectation is that service planning and delivery will take account of this. Indeed it is presented as a ten-year programme for change (DH, 2005c).

The introduction of the NSF for Long Term Conditions has been welcomed, for example: 'The national service framework for long term conditions heralds a welcome shift away from the narrow medical models of the past and, if interpreted in the right spirit, it could be a catalyst for much better care' (Agrawal and Mitchell, 2005, p. 1281) It has also been suggested that nurses, not doctors, are the key to implementing the chronic care model in a patient-centred care team. By nature of their education and role, nurses are in a position to champion the transformation of chronic care (Bodenheimer and MacGregor, 2005). The central role of case management and Community Matrons, as part of this policy response, indicates that the nursing contribution is going to be a crucial determinant of its success. This represents a major programme of work and the next section of the chapter will examine the other elements that are part of this programme, and identify the implications for nursing that arise from this approach to the care of patients with long term conditions.

Case management

There is no single model of case management, and the term is used to describe a range of approaches to improve the organization and coordination of services for people with severe and complex health problems. Many forms of case management already exist in the NHS and new arrangements are emerging. The core elements of case management are case finding or screening, assessment, care planning, implementation, monitoring and review. They may be undertaken as part of the specific job of a 'case manager' or as a series of tasks fulfilled by members of a team (Hutt et al., 2004). The intention is that this approach will help ensure the delivery of coordinated care to meet the varied and differing needs of individual clients with long term conditions. Two people who both have type 2 diabetes, heart failure and have had a stroke will require a different treatment package dependent on the severity of their illnesses, their level of family support and their individual response to their circumstances. If the broad range of long term illnesses is then considered it can be seen that there will be huge variation in the needs of patients arising from their particular condition, social situation and local service provision. The translation of national policy statements into practice is reliant on health and social care staff working in collaboration with patients and their families to achieve this individualized care; in many areas though this has become the responsibility of Community Matrons.

The Community Matron

The competencies identified for the Community Matrons add up to a formidable task (Hudson, 2005). It is one thing for policy makers to state what they would like to happen, it is quite another for that vision to become reality; particularly if, as Hudson (2005) identifies, nothing is done to address some underlying deficits in existing management systems. Although commitment was given to appoint 3,000 Community Matrons by March 2007 to 'spearhead the case management drive' (DH, 2005d) the simple arithmetic outlines the scale of the task. There are 17.5 million people with a long term condition in the United Kingdom. Approximately 3,000 Community Matrons are to be appointed with a caseload of around 50–80 patients (DH, 2005d), this amounts to 240,000 clients who will be managed by the matrons. Not every patient will require input at all times, however the extremely complex needs of a small number of individual clients could potentially occupy the Community Matrons 'full time' if genuinely individualized care is to be delivered. The comprehensive skill set that these practitioners will require (DH, 2005a), further emphasizes the challenge facing nurses who take on such roles. Also the expectation that they will work across the boundaries of health, social and voluntary care sectors is not as straightforward as may first appear. Organizations in these different sectors have different structures, procedures and traditions, which can impair cross sector working. Fully integrated health and social care teams remain the exception rather than the rule (Wilson et al., 2005). Similarly the commissioning process, which governs how services are delivered and paid for will need to be adjusted to ensure provision for people with long term conditions is adequately funded. Health Authorities have requested clearer guidelines so that they know which long term patients they are required to provide funding for and those they are not responsible for (*British Medical Journal* [BMJ], 2005). This illustrates how policy pronouncements may indicate a direction of travel, however they need to be underpinned by clear organizational and financial structures locally if they are to be implemented. Perhaps most significantly the progress in recruiting the Community Matrons has not matched the policy aspiration. Currently there are 1,348 matrons in England, less than half the target number (Primary Health Care, 2007) and this is likely to impair service delivery for patients with Long Term Conditions (LTCs) as their role is central to the policy solution that has been adopted.

Implications for nurses

The Community Matron role has been established to manage the coordination of care provision for people with long term conditions, however the delivery of that care will involve everyone in the health and social care team, particularly in view of the number of matrons being fewer than anticipated. As far back as 1984 Strauss recognized that to care for patients with chronic illnesses medical knowledge has to be supplemented with psychological and social knowledge. If this can be achieved then care is likely to improve because although different illnesses present different challenges, arising from specific symptomology and prognoses, people who are chronically ill face many similar problems (Strauss, 1984). Chronic illnesses:

- Are long term by nature
- Are uncertain
- Require palliation rather than cure
- Are multiple diseases
- Are intrusive
- Require the provision of a wide range of support services
- Are expensive. (Strauss, 1984)

To a large extent the current policy framework is an attempt to address these long standing problems in a comprehensive and structured way. This presents many implications for nursing however, and the remainder of this chapter the will focus on three areas that are clearly identified in the key policy documents: care planning, supported self-care, and longer term development.

Care planning

The guidance provided by the Department of Health (2005d) includes the following 'indicative' steps:

- Approach the patients identified as high risk and seek their agreement to be supported through case management
- Develop single comprehensive care plans which are agreed between individuals and specialist clinicians (and agencies), with all participants having a copy
- Ensure these care plans set out agreed health objectives and care needs for the person and the contributions of the individual and of each agency to meeting these
- Assess the possibility of providing self-care skills training so that the individual is able to take better care of themselves
- Ensure care plans also include arrangements for emergency or contingency arrangements.

Patient-centred care planning which addresses the diverse range of patients' needs has been a central feature of nursing for many years (Bassett and Makin, 2000; Mallett and Dougherty, 2000). On one level, these requirements would not seem to be proposing anything new. However, on closer examination the impact of these recommendations becomes clearer. Moving to a situation where the patient 'owns' his or her care plan will require changes in the working practices of all the agencies involved, as well as a move to genuine partnership working with clients. This will affect all branches of nursing. For example nurses working with children who experience birth injury will need to work with the parents, the child and all partner agencies to develop a lifelong plan of care which will require different levels of intervention at various stages in the life-course. Clients with learning difficulties are living longer and so will need sensitive care plans, which incorporate appropriate strategies for addressing their health and social care needs. In all care plans for people with long term conditions, the clear identification of 'trigger points' where increased support and care is needed is vital. For example plans will need to include a provision for support of any friend or relative who is providing on-going care, for example if this individual becomes ill. If no mechanism is in place for providing 'cover' the patient is likely to be admitted to hospital. However if the planning is effective, supplementary support in the form of a health professional or another family friend will be 'activated' and thus prevent an unnecessary admission of the patient to hospital. Similarly clients with long term mental health problems may experience acute episodes which can be managed in the community if measures are stated in the plan to address this. Inclusion of monthly assessments as part of the plan would make it possible to identify when an acute episode is imminent and appropriate action needed. A new, longer view of care will need to be adopted so that it is not thought of as a series of isolated episodes, or encounters but rather as a negotiated continuing partnership with the client.

Self-care

This view is also evident in the recommendations made concerning supported self-care (DH, 2005d). They reflect the different form care will need to take in the future in that for this client group it will be less about direct care giving by nurses and more about education and support, for example:

- Helping patients to develop the knowledge and skills they need to manage and monitor their own conditions, including providing self-care tools such as blood pressure cuffs, diets and referrals to community resources
- Ensuring clients can be actively involved, if they wish, in planning their personalized care
- Encouraging people to set goals for improving the care of their condition
- Encouraging people to form self-care support networks to provide peer support to one another

- Developing lifestyle education programmes in physical activity, healthy eating and other healthy habits.

Nurses currently undertake many of these roles in their everyday practice, however the emphasis given to this approach (DH, 2005d; 2005b) indicates that this needs to be firmly embedded in nursing if this policy imperative is to be met (also see Chapter 6 in this volume).

Finally nurses have been called upon to take the following actions, as it is believed they will help improve the care of people with long term conditions (DH, 2005e):

- Get involved in policy and planning for older people, chronic disease management and palliative care
- Challenge myths that prevent moving forward
- Involve patients in decision making and offer choice
- Look at whole population not only individuals on the caseload
- Lead for change
- Work with PCT to identify priorities and influence commissioning
- Work towards raising the profile of primary and community nursing so the public and other professionals understand roles.

These are examples of how nurses can become more involved in policy at the meso-level. As well as adapting the role of nursing to work in partnership with patients with long term conditions more is expected of them from policy makers in terms of a wider sphere of activity. It may be difficult to envisage how influence can be brought to bear on commissioning when struggling with a large caseload and working with patients, enabling them to improve their skills in self-care. However it is never too early to think about how these longer term objectives can be achieved (see below). Offering to speak for nursing on committees in consultation exercises is often a useful starting point. If this is underpinned by some leadership training and a commitment to presenting and supporting the patients' perspective a number of definite steps to policy involvement have already been taken. This is likely to become increasingly important because patients are continuing to receive intermittent, ad hoc care in response to crises, yet have little preventative intervention in between. Though many professionals are involved in their care, no one has responsibility for considering all of the patient's health and social care needs, or for ensuring they are met (DH, 2005e). The role of the Community Matron and the nurse more generally could be developed to take this central responsibility. Nurses are ideally placed to take on this role and indeed many already have. Some success has been reported in the United States (Bodenheimer and MacGregor, 2005) and the active involvement of nurses and nursing will be crucial to its success in the United Kingdom.

In a recent study Corben and Rosen (2005) reviewed the literature on self-management of long term conditions, focusing specifically on patients' perspectives. They worked with the Long Term Medical Conditions Alliance (LMCA, see below) to interview nine people living with different conditions and convened an e-conference group of six people working in the field. Although this was not an explicitly sociological study in the tradition of those referred to in Chapter 1, it gives similar emphasis to the patients' experience. They investigated patient views on how service providers should support patients to self-manage and they found a patient's encounter with a health professional will be positive if the professional:

- Has the ability to listen
- Identifies the patient's main concerns
- Allows time for discussion
- Understands how the patient experiences his/her condition
- Ensures that the patient contributes to the planning of his/her care

This is enhanced if the professional plans care *with* patients, not *for* them and is able to provide clear accessible information. They found patients want continuity of care, enough time to talk, and service planning that fits in with people's lives, including out of hours care (Corben and Rosen, 2005). These principles outline a framework for care for nurses working with people who have long term conditions that is consistent with the policy framework and the available research.

It is based on collaboration, listening and understanding, all essential elements of nursing. However when considering the role of the nurse in policy these skills need to be extended to apply to a different sphere of activity.

Longer term development

In a study investigating the relationship of policy to care of elderly people in long term care environments Tolson et al. concluded that the practice development agenda co-exists with and responds to the policy context and if the policy context is unclear or inaccessible to nurses, this may undermine development aspirations and the quality of service provision (Tolson et al., 2005). So if longer term engagement with the policy process is to occur it will require an understanding of the process outlined earlier in the chapter along with an awareness of current policy initiatives. One area where these elements come together is in 'Policy Networks'. In the context of long term conditions the (LMCA, 2005) is a policy network, sometimes referred to as a policy community, which serves to try and ensure that the care of people with long term conditions continues to attract attention, claim legitimacy and invoke action.

Policy communities are networks characterized by a defined membership which seeks to shape policy in a particular area (Rhodes and Marsh, 1992). Networks of all types consist of a set of nodes (people) linked by some form of relationships (or ties), and delineated by specific criteria (Lewis, 2005). They act at the meso-level (Hudson and Lowe, 2004) where the relationship is between interest groups and the government (Rhodes and Marsh, 1992). A number of organizations have come together in the form of the LMCA and the Partnership on Long term conditions. The LMCA is, as the name suggests, an alliance of 109 organizations including Arthritis Care, The British Heart Foundation, The Cystic Fibrosis Trust and Diabetes Care. Its aims are:

● to lobby for full implementation of existing health and social care policies that will improve the lives of people affected by long term conditions

- to influence the creation and content of new national health and social care policies, and other aspects of public policy where appropriate, to benefit people affected by long term conditions
- to promote a wide range of sustainable high quality self-management programmes for people affected by long term conditions
- to support member organizations to develop strong voices and effective services for their particular user groups
- to extend LMCA's existing work for people affected by long term conditions to benefit other health and social care service users
- to strengthen the health voluntary sector infrastructure to enable patient/carer voices to have a stronger influence on national policy making

It works towards the achievement of these aims by campaigning for change and influencing policy, through undertaking research, producing publications, managing events, conducting meetings, publicizing its work in the media, and encouraging individuals to serve as members of consultative committees and work with other organizations. Similarly the Partnership on Long term Conditions is made up of 22 organizations, including the LMCA, the NHS Confederation and a range of other organizations some of which are in the LMCA and some which are not, and has produced a 'Manifesto for Change' (Partnership on Long Term Conditions, 2005). This document itemizes what the member organizations wish to happen, in political terms. It lists a series of outcomes that are to be achieved, 'By the end of the next parliament'. This is an explicit recognition of the need to engage with the political process to ensure the needs of people with long term conditions are met. These reflect and supplement the stated targets in the NSF. For example:

- Everyone with a long term condition should receive early, accurate and expert diagnosis of their condition and assessment of their needs
- Comprehensive health information resources should offer everyone equal access to high quality health information to help them make decisions about their lives

- Such resources should be developed with voluntary organizations, taking advantage of their substantial expertise in this field
- Everyone with a long term condition should be offered a personal care plan and should be offered a choice of appropriate, convenient, and accessible lay-led self-management programmes

The role of policy networks emphasize that policy is not simply about government initiatives and actions. Groups representing and supporting people who have a range of long term conditions are actively shaping the policy response to this personal and social issue. As well as understanding the dynamics of this process, nurses can use their experience and expertise to become more involved in it.

Conclusion

It is clear that chronic disabling disorders are the major cause of mortality and present a significant challenge to the health and social care system (Locker, 1991). Although the scale and importance of this issue has been apparent for many years (Strauss and Corbin, 1988; Strauss, 1984) it has only become a significant feature on the UK Health Policy agenda relatively recently, and the reasons for this have been discussed. People are living longer, and some of those extra years are spent in ill health. Those with multiple conditions are disproportionate users of health care resources, with two thirds of emergency hospital admissions being for exacerbations of long term conditions. The policy challenge is to move away from a health care system based around acute episodes of ill health towards supporting those with long term conditions in appropriate care settings. Health care in the United Kingdom is delivered within a complex and highly political context and the consideration of this context in the chapter is intended to provide some insights on how the treatment and care of patients with long term conditions is likely to be organized for the next few years. Nurses have a central role to play in this area of service provision and an appreciation of the contribution of policy and sociological perspectives can increase our understanding of this area and ultimately assist us in providing responsive and sensitive care.

References

6, P., 'Can policy making be evidence-based?', *Managing Community Care*, 10: 1 (2002) 3–8.

Agrawal N., and A.J. Mitchell, 'The national service framework for long term conditions', *British Medical Journal*, 330: 7503 (2005) 1280–1281.

Allsop J., *Health Policy and the NHS-Towards 2000* (London: Longman, 1995).

Bassett C., and L. Makin, *Caring for the Seriously Ill Patient* (London: Arnold, 2000).

Bergen A., and A. While, ' "Implementation deficit" and "street-level bureaucracy": policy, practice and change in the development of community nursing issues', *Health and Social Care in the Community*, 13: 1 (2005) 1–10.

Bodenheimer T., and K. MacGregor, 'Nurses as leaders in chronic care', *British Medical Journal*, 330: 7492 (2005) 611–612.

Brehaut J.D., and D. Juzwishin, *Bridging the Gap: the Use of Research Evidence in Policy Development* (Alberta: Alberta Heritage Foundation for Medical Research, 2005).

British Household Panel Survey, www.iser.essex.ac.uk/ulsc/bhps (2001) (last accessed 20 December 2007).

British Medical Journal (BMJ), 'Authorities want clearer guidelines about funding long term care', *British Medical Journal*, 330 (2005) 618.

Canadian Health Services Research Foundation, 'Interdisciplinary teams in primary healthcare can effectively manage chronic illness', *Evidence Boost September* 2005, http://www.chsrf. ca/mythbusters/pdf/boost3_e.pdf (2005) 1–2 (last accessed 20 December 2007).

Corben S., and S. Rosen, *Self-Management for Long-Term Conditions: Patients' Perspectives on the Way Ahead* (London: King's Fund, 2005).

Crinson I., 'The direction of health policy in New Labour's third term', *Critical Social Policy*, 25: 4 (2005) 507–516.

Davies H.T.O., S.M. Nutley and P.C. Smith, 'Editorial: what works? The role of evidence in public sector policy and practice', *Public Money & Management*, 19: 1 (1999) 3–5.

Department of Health (DH), *The Expert Patient Programme: a New Approach to Chronic Disease Management for the 21st Century* (London: DH, 2001).

Department of Health (DH), 10 *High Impact Changes for Service Improvement and Delivery: A Guide for NHS Leaders* (Leicester: DH, 2004a).

Department of Health (DH), *National Standards, Local Action – Health and Social Care Standards and Planning Framework 2005/6–2007/8* (London: DH, 2004b).

Department of Health/NHS Modernisation Agency and Skills for Health, *Case Management and Competencies Framework for the Care of People with Long Term Conditions* (London: DH, 2005a).

Department of Health (DH), *Choosing Health* (London: DH, 2005b).

Department of Health (DH), *The National Service Framework for Long-Term Conditions* (London: DH, 2005c).

Department of Health (DH), *Supporting People with Long Term Conditions* (4230) (London: DH, 2005d).

Department of Health (DH), *Supporting People with Long Term Conditions Liberating the Talents of Nurses Who Care for People with Long Term Conditions* (3853) (London: DH, 2005e).

General Household Survey www.statistics.gov.uk/ssd/surveys/ general_household_survey.asp. (2001) (last accessed 20 December 2007).

Green J., and N. Thorogood, *Analysing Health Policy – a Sociological Approach* (London: Longman, 1998).

Greener I., 'The three moments of New Labour's health policy discourse', *Policy & Politics*, 32: 3 (2004) 303–316.

Groves T., and E.H. Wagner, 'High quality care for people with chronic diseases', *British Medical Journal*, 330: 7492 (2005) 609–610.

Ham C., *Health Policy in Britain*, 5th edn (Houndmills: Palgrave Macmillan, 2004).

Ham C., 'Preface', in D. Singh, *Transforming Chronic Care: Evidence about Improving Care of People with Long-Term Conditions* (Birmingham: Health Service Management Centre, University of Birmingham, 2005a).

Ham C., 'Lost in translation? Health systems in the US and the UK', *Social Policy and Administration*, 39: 2 (2005b) 192–209.

Ham C., and M. Hill, *The Policy Process in the Modern Capitalist State* (New York: Harvester Wheatsheaf, 1993).

Hart C., *Nurses and Politics: the Impact of Power and Practice* (Houndmills: Palgrave Macmillan, 2004).

Hennessy D., 'The emerging themes', in D. Hennessy and P. Spurgeon (eds), *Health Policy and Nursing: Influence, Development and Impact* (Houndmills: Palgrave Macmillan, 2000).

Hudson B., 'Sea change or quick fix? Policy on long-term conditions in England', *Health and Social Care in the Community*, 13: 4 (2005) 378–385.

Hudson J., and S. Lowe, *Understanding the Policy Process* (Bristol: The Policy Press, 2004).

Hulme R., 'Policy transfer and the Internationalisation of social policy', *Social Policy & Society*, 4: 4 (2005) 417–425.

Hunter D.J., *Public Health Policy* (Cambridge: Polity, 2003).

Hutt R., and R. Rosen, 'A chronic case of mismanagement?' *Journal of Health Service Research and Policy*, 10: 4 (2005) 194–195.

Hutt R., R. Rosen and J. McCauley, *Case-Managing Long-Term Conditions: What Impact Does It Have in the Treatment of Older People?* (London: King's Fund, 2004).

Kingdon J.W., *Agendas, Alternatives and Public Policies* (Boston, MA: Little Brown, 1984).

Lewis J.M., 'Being around and knowing the player: networks of influence in health policy', *Social Science & Medicine*, 62 (2005) 2125–2136.

Locker D., 'Living with chronic Illness', in G. Scambler (ed.), *Sociology as Applied to Medicine* (London: Balliere Tindall, 1991).

Long Term Medical Conditions Alliance (LMCA), *Annual Review* (London: LMCA, 2005).

Mallet J., and L. Doughtery, *The Royal Marsden Manual of Clinical Nursing Procedures*, 5th edn (Oxford: Blackwell Science, 2000).

Masterson A., 'Cross-boundary working: a macro-political analysis of the impact on professional roles', *Journal of Advanced Nursing*, 11: 3 (2002) 331–339.

Masterson B., 'What is social policy?', in P. Gough, S. Maslin-Prothero and A. Masterson (eds), *Nursing and Social Policy* (Oxford: Butterworth Heinemann, 1994).

Partnership on Long-term Conditions, *17 Millions Reasons: Improving the Lives of People with Long-Term Conditions*. Partnership on Long-term Conditions, 2005, http://www.17millionreasons.co.uk/Downloads/Chron_disease_manifesto_V7.pdf (last accessed 12 September 2008).

Primary Health Care, 'Number of community matrons is less than half of government promise' (news item), 17: 3 (2007) www.nursing-standard.co.uk/primaryhealthcare/news2.asp (last accessed 20 December 2007).

Rhodes R.A., and D. Marsh (1992) 'Policy networks in British politics. A critique of existing approaches', in D. Marsh and R.A.W. Rhodes (eds), *Policy Networks in British Government* (Oxford: Oxford University Press, 1992).

Singh D., *Transforming Chronic Care: Evidence about Improving Care of People with Long-Term Conditions* (Birmingham: Health Service Management Centre, University of Birmingham, 2005).

Solesbury W., 'The environmental agenda', *Public Administration,* Winter (1976) 379–397.

South Birmingham Primary Care Trust, PCT Board Meeting Minutes 13 September, Agenda Item 14 (Enclosure 11) (2006) www.Southbirminghampct.nhs.uk/board/2006/cnl11 (last accessed 16 October 2006).

Strauss A., and J.M. Corbin, *Shaping a New Health Care System* (San Francisco: Jossey-Bass Publishers, 1988).

Strauss A.L., *Chronic Illness and the Quality of Life* (St Louis: Mosby, 1984).

Tolson D., W. Maclaren, S. Kieley and A. Lowndes, 'Influence of policies on nursing practice in long-term care environments for older people', *Journal of Advanced Nursing,* 50: 6 (2005) 661–671.

Walshe K., 'The rise of regulation in the NHS', *British Medical Journal,* 324 (2002) 967–970.

Walt G., *Health Policy – an Introduction to Policy and Power* (London: Zed Books, 1994).

Wanless D., J. Appleby, A. Harrison and D. Patel, *Our Future Health Secured? a Review of NHS Funding and Performance* (London: King's Fund, 2007).

West E., and C. Scott, 'Nursing in the public sphere: breaching the boundary between research and policy', *Journal of Advanced Nursing,* 32: 4 (2000) 817–824.

Wilson T., D. Buck and C. Ham, 'Rising to the challenge: will the NHS support people with long term conditions?', *British Medical Journal,* 330: 7492 (2005) 657–661.

3 Researching people with long term conditions

Gayle Letherby

Introduction

In this chapter I consider issues of method, methodology and epistemology relevant to researching about, with and for people with long term conditions. The methods we choose and our methodological experiences are influenced by the topic under investigation. Furthermore the research process itself influences the research product. Researching people with long term conditions may suggest particular methods and militate against the use of others. Our methodological approach to research and experience of the research process may also be tempered by the disability and/or chronic illness of the respondent group. Issues of power, emotion, sensitivity, involvement and detachment are relevant here, as in all research, as is the acknowledgement of difference and diversity and of research praxis.

Bowling provides a useful overview of the types of research focusing on health and health services:

> Research on health and health services ranges from descriptive investigations of the experience of illness and people's perceptions of health and ill health...to evaluation of health services in relation to their appropriateness, effectiveness and costs...However, these two areas overlap and should not be rigidly divided, as it is essential to include the perspective of the lay person in health service evaluation and decision-making. Other related fields of investigation include audit, quality assurance, and the assessments of needs for health services (usually defined in terms of the need for effective services), which comes within the umbrella of health research but also has a crucial link with health services research. (Bowling, 2002, p. 6)

Research about the experience of living with a long term condition includes both health research and health services research.

In this chapter, my concern is with how social researchers measure and understand the social and medical experience of people with long term conditions. The focus in on issues of method (the tools for data gathering: e.g. questionnaires, interviews, conversational analysis), of methodology (the analysis of the methods used) and of epistemology (the theory of knowledge). People new to research may be forgiven for thinking that this chapter is one to skip over before getting to the more interesting ones about actual examples and experiences of long term conditions. But, social researchers (and physical scientists and health researchers), need to be clear about their motivations for research, their methods of data collection and how the research process affects the research product (the findings, and the theoretical pronouncements). Thus, any account of research focusing on the experience of long term conditions, just like any account of research, should include some reference to the research process.

Choosing ...

The methods that social scientists use can broadly be classified into quantitative methods (those that involve the collection and analysis of numbers) and qualitative methods (involving collection, observation and analysis of words and actions). Both quantitative and qualitative researchers collect and analyze primary data (data collected for the current research project) and secondary data (already existing documents and artifacts).

Examples of quantitative data collection involving primary methods are surveys (which include self-completed questionnaires) and structured interviews (which provide respondents with a limited range of questions and responses). Quantitative secondary data might include hospital or public records and previously administered and analyzed questionnaires which can all be (re)analyzed by the researcher. Using quantitative research methods, we can measure the frequency of particular conditions and attitudes towards them – everything from childhood cancer to anorexia. Quantitative research methods also allow us to measure the amount of interaction between patient and practitioner. Following this we can make comparisons between the experience of individuals who suffer from long term conditions and those who have more acute conditions. Comparisons are also possible between and within specific conditions with reference to socio-economic, gender, age and other differences.

Historically quantitative methods were deemed to be 'scientific' and unquestioned as the best way to study both the natural and the social world. From this perspective the view is that the 'expert neutral knower' (the researcher) can be separated from what is known; that different researchers exposed to the same data can replicate results and that it is possible to generalize from research to wider social and natural populations. In other words the 'scientific' method allows for the 'objective' collection of facts by a value-neutral researcher (Letherby, 2003; Stanley and Wise, 1993). Those that aim for a 'scientific' social science argue that the research process is linear and orderly (Kelly et al., 1994; Stanley and Wise, 1993). This approach is generally known as positivism and associated with quantitative methods (but it is important to remember that not all quantitative researchers are aiming for positivism/a 'scientific' approach. See Oakley, 1999 for further discussion). Challenging the traditional 'scientific' approach with specific reference to research with disabled people (but her point is generalizable), Stalker argues:

> ...conventional research relationships, whereby the researcher is the 'expert' and the researched merely the object of investigation, are inequitable;...people have the right to be consulted about and involved in the research which is concerned with issues affecting their lives;...the quality and relevance of research is improved when disabled people are closely involved in the process. (Stalker, 1998, p. 6)

There has been and is much criticism of the use of numbers to 'prove facts' in social life and qualitative methods are often seen as a response/critique to the so-called scientific approach. Qualitative methods focus on the 'experiential' in the belief that the best way to find out about people is to let them 'speak for themselves' (Stanley and Wise, 1993). The use of qualitative research is also seen by some as a way of giving respondents more control over the research process. Qualitative researchers then are concerned to generate data grounded in the experience of respondents. Qualitative primary methods include single, dyad and focus group interviews, participant and non-participant observation, exchange of letters and respondent diary keeping whilst documents and artefacts such as letters and diaries (not written for the purpose of the research), photographs and medical texts are all subject to secondary analysis. Qualitative methods focus on experience rather than measurement and so (for example) instead of the amount of interaction between practitioner and patient the qualitative researcher would be interested in the meanings of the interactions (Sharp, 2005). On first reflection qualitative methods might appear to be the most appropriate to use when researching long term conditions. As Koch and Kralik argue while writing about their research focusing on the experience of living with chronic illness:

> Story telling has engaged researcher attention as a method of accessing the personal world of illness... For the purpose of our enquiries, verbal accounts are more than vehicles for collecting personal information; they are the very processes of identity construction. Asking people to tell their story of chronic illness is the most appropriate way to explore how identity is constructed when people are in 'transition'. (Koch and Kralik, 2001, p. 34)

But it is important not to rule out other methods and approaches. As with many other research areas flexibility is necessary (for further discussion, see Kelly et al., 1994; Letherby and Zdrodowski, 1995; Reinharz, 1992; Stanley and Wise, 1993). Critiquing what she calls the 'paradigm wars', Oakley (1998, p. 709) argues that there is a danger that quantitative and qualitative approaches are represented as 'mutually exclusive ideal types'. Cautioning against choosing favourite methods without proper consideration of the research aims and objectives Kelly et al. (1994) argue that appropriate methods should be chosen to suit research programmes rather than research programmes being chosen to 'fit' favourite techniques. In addition, Oakley (2004, p. 191) suggests: 'The most important criteria for choosing a particular research method is not its relationship to academic arguments about methods, but its fit with the question being asked in the research'. Kelly et al., add: 'Rather than assert the primacy of any method, we are not working with a flexible position: our choice of method(s) depends on the topic and scale of the study in question. Whenever possible we would combine and compare methods, in order to discover the limitations and possibilities of each' (Kelly et al., 1994, p. 35–36).

Note similar warnings not to perpetuate an artificial divide between the quantitative and the qualitative and to combine the best of different methods by The National Science Foundation:

> ...a quantitative/qualitative divide permeates much of social science, but this should be seen as a continuum rather than a dichotomy. At the one end of this continuum is textbook quantitative research marked by sharply defined and delineated populations, cases and variables, and well specified theoretical hypotheses. At the opposite of this continuum is social research that eschews notions of populations, cases and variables altogether and rejects the possibility of hypotheses testing...In between these two extremes are many different research strategies including many hybrid and combined strategies. (The National Science Foundation, 2004, p. 9)

Thus, mixed method research, multi-method research, methodological pluralism or as it is sometimes called triangulation (which can include not only a combination of different methods but also/or a combination of methodological positions or theoretical viewpoints) is often the most desirable way to undertake research. This can include a mixture of the quantitative (such as a study using a questionnaire focusing on waiting lists and waiting times and a review of hospital records recording the same data) or the qualitative (as in an ethnographic study of a outpatients clinic involving non-participant observation, interviews and analysis of patient notes) or some combination of quantitative and qualitative methods (Miller and Brewer, 2003).

Starting ...

Research in the area of long term conditions might be being undertaken as part of undergraduate or postgraduate study, or may be the result of a successful grant application or research tender. Projects may be conducted by individual researchers, by single discipline research teams or by multi-discipline and multi-agency groups. Once the research and basic project aims and objectives are defined one of the first things that the researcher(s) have to do is obtain ethical approval. Depending on both the institutional base of the researcher(s) and the research site and population, this may be a multi-tiered process. Thus, for a project on out-reach support for individuals with mental health conditions it may be necessary for a researcher to obtain ethical approval from their university ethics committee, from a locally based external ethics board that vets all projects that involve health professionals, patients or patient records and from the management committees/trustees of various charities and self-help groups. In addition most discipline areas have their own research ethics guidelines that influence research design and research process.

The benefits of taking ethical issues seriously are obvious and include providing confidentiality for respondents, taking regard of health and safety issues for respondents and researchers and meeting obligations to research funders during the research process. However, ethics are not just about individual 'good behaviour' and the concern with research ethics has been influenced by the drive for greater user involvement and protection of respondents as well as the development and maintenance of professional integrity in the research process (Letherby and Bywaters, 2007). A key concern of ethics committee is that of informed consent that is that respondents are consenting to involvement in research from a position of full understanding. Yet, it is usually difficult to assess whether consent is 'really' informed:

> Dilemmas include; the value of signed consent forms; how to assess the ability (or 'competence') of individuals to give informed consent, especially for groups characterized as 'vulnerable'; how to recognise that people want to withdraw from their involvement in a research study; how to avoid gatekeepers denying consent for people to participate or including people who have not truly consented; and whether consent should be restricted to data collection or include the ways that data are interpreted and presented. (Wiles et al., 2005, p. 3)

This is just one indication that ethics committees are not the guardians of research ethics that they hope to be. Others include the fact that they do not allow for change and development within the research process:

> A condition of ethical approval being granted, is that [the research ethics committee] ask to be informed of any changes to the research protocol.... Research methodology is often required to change once

research participants become part of the research process, yet the relationship of [research ethics committees] to research processes means that some researchers may be reluctant to re-enter the ethical approval process once initial approval has been withdrawn; secondly, the bureaucratic nature of [research ethics committees] means that they are not able to respond in a timely or constructive way to genuine ethical concerns which unfold during the course of a study. For this to happen, there needs to be 'a shift in our common-sense understanding of ethics as a property of individuals who monadically reflect on dilemmas.... it requires a much broader set of activities than is associated with conventional professional ethics' (Rossiter et al., 2000, p. 95). (Truman, 2003, p. 3.25)

And on occasion they do not understand the particular research design and methodology that the researcher is proposing:

In October 1995, I began a PhD that looked at women's experiences of living with coronary heart disease ... At that time, the majority of the ethics committee were consultant physicians and surgeons. All submissions (unless submitted by medical consultants) were required to have a sponsor... since I aimed to have a nursing focus in my research, I chose the only senior nurse from the Trust who had the background to fulfill the sponsor's role...

I still have the letter sent by the committee administrator. Six years on, the comments continue to arouse feelings of horror and humour. They revealed that a number of the committee members were totally ignorant about qualitative research. ... The main areas of concern were that the study only included women, had a qualitative methodology and that there was a potential for researcher bias ...

The committee's second concern was with the qualitative nature of the study. Three members simply viewed qualitative research as unethical. Comments were made about the hypothesis (there was no hypothesis), the lack of a control group and the poor experimental design. One member commented: 'This submission looks like bad science and therefore is not to be supported on ethical grounds'. I responded to this by highlighting the fact that qualitative research was methodologically and ethically sound and that prestigious medical journals regularly publish the results of qualitative research. (from a vignette by Lockyer in Hallowell et al., 2005, pp. 72–82)

As part of the ethical approval process researchers need to indicate the characteristics of their proposed respondent group and how they will access them. Research involving gatekeepers and/or translators (i.e., people other than respondents) may discourage respondents who feel that these others may then have access to what they have divulged through the course of the research. Arguably, this is particularly relevant when researching people who are receiving support, care or treatment as they may worry that what they say will influence future support/care/treatment which may, in turn and when relevant affect their treatment and their care from these individuals (Afshar, 1994; Cannon, 1989). Gatekeeping issues are also relevant when trying to research respondents in the private sphere, and when researching personal and family issues as individuals may not want other family members to know all the specifics of a condition or the emotions surrounding it (Exley and Letherby, 2001). Further complications may arise when the researcher and some, or all, of the respondent group do not speak the same language, when respondents are children or have a physical condition or learning disability which is likely to involve them telling their story through another (see, for example, Afshar and Maynard, 1994 and Hood et al., 1999).

Whilst recruitment and data collection which necessitates the involvement of 'others' can be problematic, so too can be recruitment and data collection with self-selecting, self-identifying respondents. For my own research on 'infertility' and 'involuntary childlessness', (I write 'infertility' and 'involuntary childlessness' in single quotation marks to highlight the problems of definition.) I advertized for individuals who defined themselves at that time or some time in the past as 'infertile' and/or 'involuntarily childless'. This recruitment method meant that I had people come forward who I did not define in the same way. In addition, self-selection as a recruitment method clearly has an influence on the data in that it affects what respondents say and how they say it. In my research, those who did not come forward but would have been willing to be involved if accessed through an 'infertility' clinic or adoption support group were likely to have had different things to say. Many of my respondents had clear political motivations 'to put the record straight', 'to tell it how it is'. The same was true of the respondents in the research of Kralik et al.,:

Women were invited to participate in the study in several ways. Women joined the study by responding to an article placed in the reader's pages of a widely distributed Australian woman's magazine.

Short articles were also placed in the newsletters of organizations established to support people who live with long-term illness. The newsletter of one support group was placed on the Internet, and that resulted in participants from many parts of the world joining the study. Several women who were participating in the study also recruited other participants. *There was no difficulty in attracting women to participate. On the contrary, many women commented that for a long time they had wanted to be heard because they had so many stories to tell.* (Kralik et al., 2000, p. 912, my emphasis)

In my research and in that by Kralik et al. (2000), others for whom their condition was less of an issue or for whom the issues were 'too painful' to share were less well represented (Letherby, 2003). Attention to issues of difference and diversity extend beyond the inclusion (or exclusion) of people with different experiences and viewpoints of the same condition and it is necessary to pay attention to the social characteristics (age, sex, 'race', sexuality, etc.) of respondents. Some individuals and groups may be harder to reach and accessing less represented and minority populations can be expensive in terms of both financial and temporal resources (Cannon et al., 1991; Letherby and Bywaters, 2007; Standing, 1998).

An additional concern during the beginning stages of a project may be the formation of an advisory or steering group. This may be a condition of approval by either external ethics boards and/or funders/commissioners or an original concern of the research team. Steering group members can act as advisors, as sounding boards, as providers of local and other knowledge, as representatives of interest groups, as resources for respondents, as critics of interim reports and ongoing data analysis, and as allies in the presentation and publication of the research findings. Funders or commissioners may identify members, with the researcher(s) having little or no involvement in the process; alternatively, researchers may work independently or with funders/commissioners to identify appropriate people. Increasingly steering groups consist of service users as well as professionals although it can prove difficult to involve lay people or groups in steering groups for a variety of reasons: lack of interest, lack of time, lack of resources and personal ill-health (Letherby and Bywaters, 2007; Scott et al., 1999).

Doing ...

Having designed the project, obtained ethical approval, accessed respondents and, if appropriate, held an initial meeting with the research steering group the research can begin. Yet, the need for flexibility and sensitivity is far from over. Problems and dilemmas are endemic to the whole research process and in recent years the research experience has itself become an issue of concern:

> When we enter a field we make footprints on the land and are likely to disturb the environment. When we leave we may have mud on our shoes, pollen on our clothes. If we leave the gate open this may have serious implications for the farmers and their animals. All of this is also relevant to what we find out about the field and its inhabitants. Thus, when doing research (fieldwork) we need to be sensitive to respondents and to the relevance to our own presence in their lives and in the research process. (Letherby, 2003, p. 6)

This indicates the need for researchers to be aware of their own personal and intellectual personhood and its significance to both the research process and product. Acknowledgement of this is necessary if the knowledge produced is to be 'accountable' (Stanley, 1991). Hallowell et al. (2005) note that authors are more willing than ever to acknowledge that empirical research, and in particular qualitative research, is what Bryne-Armstrong et al. (2001, p. vii) have called a 'complex, often chaotic, sometimes messy, even conflictual' endeavour. However they add 'despite what could be called the "reflexive turn" in research reporting, the realities of doing empirical research are generally glossed over in methods textbooks, research reports and journal articles, which still provide fairly sanitized accounts of the research process' (Hallowell et al., 2005, p. 2).

This is a shame for all social research is chaotic and messy, not least because it involves human beings whose lives are at times chaotic and messy also. In addition, there are no 'blueprints' for social research and for many respondents the questionnaire they complete, the reflective diary they write or the focus group they attend may be their first experience of research. As noted earlier, it is difficult to fully inform respondents of all there is to know about research. (After all, it takes researchers many years to qualify and the learning process continues beyond graduation.) Complications can arise when respondents assume that the research will result in better immediate support or treatment for them or when they perceive the researcher as 'expert', as 'counsellor', as 'kindred spirit' or indeed in any role other than that as data collector (Collins, 1998; Cotterill and Letherby, 1994). I am not saying here that researchers and respondents do not adopt 'roles' and 'relationships' during the research process, merely highlighting that the inevitable positioning of researcher and respondent does have consequences for the research. The research process is a complex endeavour, and the researcher's status as 'insider' and 'outsider' may be subject to constant negotiation between all parties. A researcher's 'insider' status may be assumed by the respondent and/or the researcher if the researcher shares an identity or experience with respondents or works with similar others in a professional capacity, as colleague or carer. One example here is the nurse-nurse researcher who could be argued to be experiencing role conflict (Colbourne, 2004).

Such involvement is often thought to lead to bias on behalf of the researcher but as I and others have suggested issues of self and other are always a part of research and thus should always be reflected upon (Fine, 1994; Wilkinson and Kitzinger, 1996; Temple, 1997; Letherby, 2003; Colbourne, 2004). With specific reference to the nurse researcher Linda Colbourne (2004) argues that drawing on the interactive skills of the nurse can benefit rather than detract the researcher from the research process. The researcher's identity as 'outsider', as 'stranger' rather than as 'insider' can also lead to assumptions by the researched. Thus, as Wilkinson and Kitzinger (1996, p. 18) point out that 'our work should not be so much about the other as about the interplay between the researcher and the other'.

Issues of power are complex within research and increasingly researchers are concerned with challenging a balance of power in favour of the researcher. One way to do this is through careful choice of methods and approaches. For example, Koch et al. (1999) in their study concerned with how people with type II diabetes incorporated chronic illness into their lives adopted a Participatory Action – Orientated Research (PAR). They followed Stringer's (1996) four guiding principles of PAR as:

- democratic, enabling participation of all people;
- equitable, acknowledging people's equality of worth;
- liberating, providing freedom from oppressive, debilitating conditions;
- life enhancing, enabling the expression of people's full human potential

And they argued that:

> We envisaged a community-based action research programme that sought to challenge the social and personal dynamics of the research situation and enhance the lives of all those who participated. One other important justification for us to use a PAR approach was that the principles are closely aligned to the primary health care (PHC) concepts of collaboration and empowerment. Primary health care emphasizes the participation of people in the planning and development of their own health care, and this is an important foundation for our evidence-based community nursing practice...(Koch et al., 1999, p. 27)

Similarly, Kralik et al. (2000), who, as noted earlier, researched the impact of chronic illness on the lives of midlife women, used correspondence as a method of data collection and they exchanged letters (via email and postal services) with 80 women for 12 months. This method, Kralik et al. (2000, p. 913) argue, enabled each woman to 'make sense of her thoughts and experiences through the reliving and retelling of them'. In addition research by correspondence, rather like a home-completed questionnaire, also enables the respondent to answer questions and respond to the researchers' concerns in their 'own time' rather than one determined by the researcher (Kralik et al., 2000; Letherby and Zdrodowski, 1995). It is important to note though that methods and approaches that attempt to be more inclusive, more 'respondent focused' tend to demand more resources – more time, more energy, more researchers even – and not all researchers/research teams will have access to such resources.

So, although there is an assumption that the researcher is always in control of the research situation and is the one who holds the balance of power it is often more complicated than this in reality. With this in mind it is important not to over-passify research respondents, not least by assuming that they are always vulnerable within research. Some respondents do not feel disempowered by either their life experience or by the research relationship and it may be patronizing of the researcher to assume that the respondent needs to be empowered by the process (Letherby, 2003). Respondents also have the right to be uncooperative as Davis found when researching children with multiple impairments (Davis et al., 2000). After being immersed in the research site for some time he realized that although he had assumed that 'Scott' was unable to communicate, this respondent had actually chosen not to. All research relationships are fluid and jointly constructed and at times during the research process it is the researcher that might feel vulnerable and/or at a disadvantage. This may be the case when researching individuals who are older, more experienced, more knowledgeable and/or when undertaking research with people with sexist, racist, homophobic (and so on) views and attitudes (e.g., Collins, 1998; Cotterill, 1992). People in more powerful positions – health and social care professionals for example – are likely to have more power throughout the whole research process and there are many examples of researchers being kept waiting long periods, having their methods and concerns challenged and their research agenda ignored by 'important' people (see the vignette by Ettorre in Hallowell et al., 2005 for a medical example).

Despite careful attention to research plans some respondents may be excluded along the way, not least because of issues relating to their condition as in research by Kralik et al. (see above):

Research which uses correspondence for data generation, requires that participants be literate and physically able to correspond. One woman with multiple sclerosis was unable to continue her participation in this research, as it became increasingly difficult for her to write. Another woman had received head injuries as a result of an accident and was unable to make much sense when she wrote, but may have been better able to verbally express herself. Exclusion of these women may be viewed as a disadvantage of the pen pal method. (Kralik et al., 2000, p. 913)

In an attempt to research young people with learning difficulties Booth and Booth (1996, p. 65) advocate the use of unorthodox methods saying that 'the only way of collecting their stories is to lend them the words'. As Lewis and Kellett (2004, p. 199) suggest this 'putting words into mouths...rings ethical alarm bells' but as they add 'constructing a narrative via sensitive interpretation' is likely to be more valid than less informed observations. Furthermore, as Stacey (1991, p. 144) notes, because in (almost) all research it is researchers and not respondents who hold the balance of power 'elements of inequality, exploitation, and even betrayal are endemic to [research]'.

It must be clear by now that in addition to issues of power, emotion is also an inevitable part of the research relationship/fieldwork experience (Ramsay, 1996; Young and Lee, 1996). Burkitt (1997) suggests that emotions are not internal to the individual but are found within relationships, and further to this are constituted and reconstituted in ongoing relational practices one example of this being the way in which the display of emotions is gendered. Thus, it is less acceptable for women to display stereotypical masculine emotions such as anger and less acceptable for men to display stereotypical feminine emotions such as distress (Hochschild, 1990). When reflecting on their experience of living with long term conditions male and female respondents may additionally feel hampered by social taboos and stigma attached to the/their experience. Displays of emotion with research can be dangerous for both researcher and respondent and provide another example of the need to be concerned with researcher (as well as respondent) safety and wellbeing:

> Mrs S was a twitchy participant, becoming highly animated to the point of belligerence. She smoked throughout the interview. Her answers were disconcerting and contradictory. When I asked about her family relationships, she told me that she had a good relationship with her husband. She went on to say: 'I threw a cup of tea at him this morning because he wouldn't get up'. I became increasingly nervous when she admitted that 'yes' she did have a temper...
>
> ... the part of the interview that I found most chilling was in response to my questions about her friendships. Mrs S said that she kept herself to herself, but told me that she had at one time been friendly with one neighbour but that was all over now. Mrs S no longer trusted the woman and became suspicious of her to the point where she believed the neighbour wanted to harm her. She leaned towards me

confidentially: 'She is trying to poison me by putting ground glass in my tea'. (from Alice Lovell's vignette about aspects of her research experience when studying women's health and their personal relationships, in Hallowell et al., 2005, pp. 118–119)

Building on the work of Hochschild (1983) 'emotion work' has been defined as both the regulation and managing of others' feelings and the work individuals do on their own emotions in order to conform to dominant expectations in a given situation. Thus, emotion work is work on and for others and on and for oneself (Duncombe and Marsden, 1998; Frith and Kitzinger, 1998). Furthermore, Nicky James (1989) argues that the result of the gender division of labour is that men are held responsible for bringing in the income and women for the routine running of the home and the care of children, and within this allotted role women are primarily responsible for 'working with emotions'. Ironically, given the historical focus on the so-called scientific model women researchers have traditionally been portrayed as 'more accessible and less threatening than men' which coupled with their 'superior' communicative abilities has thought to make the interactions of fieldwork generally easier (Warren, 1988, p. 45). This denies the hard work that all researchers do and is also clearly sexist.

Some writers suggest that emotion work can lead to a lack of authenticity with individuals denying their real feelings (Duncombe and Marsden, 1998; Hochschild, 1990). However, examples from my own research on the experience of 'infertility' and 'involuntary childlessness' and that of Exley's on individuals living with a terminal diagnosis suggests that individuals may engage in emotion work in their everyday lives in an attempt to maintain their authentic selves in the context of lifecourse disruption (Exley and Letherby, 2001). With this in mind it is possible to suggest that the emotion work of respondents within the research process adds to rather than detracts from a positive sense of self.

Finishing …

Analysis is not something that happens once all of the data is collected but is an ongoing part of the fieldwork process.

For this reason the 'scientific' approach to social research has been criticized not only for its unrealistic and limited view of data collected (as neutral and value-free), but also for its focus on theory-testing, or deductivism. One response was the development of grounded theory. Grounded theory is theory developed from data and aims to be faithful to the reality of situations (Strauss and Corbin, 1990). From this perspective the researcher does not begin with a theory and then prove it but allows the relevant theory to emerge from the data. However, no study can be completely inductive in the way that this approach suggests as researchers begin the research with their own political and theoretical assumptions. With this in mind it is important to remember that all research accounts are partial and constructed by the researcher. This is not to say that research reports are merely constructions but they are influenced the ideological position of the researcher(s) and their social and material location. So, as Stanley and Wise (1990, p. 22) argue 'researchers cannot have "empty heads" in the way that inductivism proposes' so one must acknowledge the gendered, classes, racial and so on intellectual and physical presence of the researcher. Thus, the personhood of the researcher is relevant to theoretical analysis just as it is to research design and fieldwork:

> Researchers are themselves people, with their own 'responses, values, beliefs, and prejudices' (Morley, 1996, p. 139) and research involves selection, explanation, interpretation and judgment. Thus, it is important that the 'person' is made explicitly and the processes involved in research procedures are clearly outlined in order to uncover the differences that we as researchers make (Jones 1997). (Letherby, 2002, p. 55)

Reflexivity – both descriptive (the description of one's reflection) and analytical (involving comparison and evaluation) – are essential parts of the research process. Furthermore, both researchers and respondents engage in it. But, it is possible to acknowledge that as researchers we are in a privileged position, not only in terms of access to multiple accounts, but also in terms of discipline training which enables us to engage in 'second order theorising' or what Giddens (1984) calls the 'double hermeneutic'. This involves 'interpretation', not just 'description' of respondents' as well as the researchers' analytical processes (Letherby, 2002).

Those who work for an emancipatory model of social research argue that in order to be ethically sound and non-exploitative research should be 'for' rather than 'of' those that are studied. An example of a research project that could be described as 'of' rather than 'for' that I have used in previous writing is particularly relevant in terms of researching long term conditions:

> [Oakley] cites a large research project on the social origins of depression by Brown and Harris (1976) and notes that the study resulted in a convincing explanation of the relationship between depression and the life events and socioeconomic circumstances. But no connection was made between women's depression and their oppression. There was no concern whether or how women defined themselves as depressed, but only with how the state of women's mental health could be exposed and fit into a system of classification developed by a profession of 'experts' on mental health (psychiatrists). Also, the researchers did not begin with a desire to study the situation of women or set out to give women a chance to understand their experience as determined by the social structure of the society in which they lived. The primary aim of the data was to study depression and women were selected as respondents because they are easier (and therefore cheaper) to interview, being more likely than men to be at home and therefore available during the day. (Letherby, 2003, p. 74)

Some researchers have agued that in order to avoid, or at least minimize, the exploitative aspects of research researchers should think carefully about attempting to represent 'others': people that are not like them. Oliver (1997), for example, suggests that some research by non-disabled people violates the experience of disabled people and is irrelevant to their needs. However, there are problems here, not least because academia is not representative of all groups; in relation to gender, ethnicity, age, dis/ability and so on, which could mean that the experience of some groups remains unconsidered (Letherby, 2003). Speaking only for ourselves could also lead to much more research on already privileged groups and implies that those who come from unrepresented and/or minority groups have a 'duty' to represent 'others' like them. It also denies criticisms of the more powerful and privileged (Letherby, 2003; Wilkinson and Kitzinger, 1996).

The use of social science knowledge for both understanding and transforming social policies and political systems has come to be assumed as demonstrated in the current emphasis of evidence-based practice (David, 2002; Solesbury, 2001). For example in Britain the Labour Governments of 1997 and 2001 have been particularly pressing in their call for evidence to support policy development, the delivery of policy objectives and the evaluation of policy outcomes. 'Good government is thinking government ... rational thought is impossible without good evidence ... social science research is central to the development and evaluation of policy' (Blunkett, 2000, p. 4). But it is important to highlight the limitations as well as the advantages of such an approach. Thus:

> Evidence-based movements are founded on the principle of raising awareness of research findings that could improve services or decision making, and ensuring that these findings are acted upon. In short, the aim is to improve research impact. This in turn has generated another layer of research and debate concerned with how best to improve research impact. (Locock and Boaz, 2004, p. 378)

In addition, it is important to remember that: ... policy makers might like to believe practitioners want the same as them, but practitioners themselves may want very different things from research, and may view research which they see as serving government interests with suspicion' (Locock and Boaz, 2004, p. 378, see also Packwood, 2002).

As Mayall et al. (1999) note, research involves three intersecting interests: those of researchers, of research respondents and of those individuals, groups and institutions with the power to influence research priorities through funding, policy making and other processes. They add that researchers have a moral obligation to take into account the impact of their work on others. Given that 'People living with chronic illness conditions are the prime health concern of the twenty first century and will remain so for the foreseeable future' (Koch and Krakik, 2001, p. 23), research on long term conditions has political implications not least in terms of the allocation of resources and the practice of professionals. In addition research in this area raises particular issues that add to our understanding of the political nature of the research process from the choice of method through to the publication of the final report.

If, as a recognition of research focusing on long term conditions as political suggests, we want our research to 'make a difference' as researchers we also need to think beyond the traditionally defined boundaries of social research. Yet despite the concern with research informed practice many if not most research texts pay little attention to non-academic publication. Furthermore, research training seldom focuses on working with the media, presentations for non-academic audiences or the representation of findings through drama. This implies the need for increased attention to the end stages of the research process, but 'extending social research' in this way likely requires attention right at the beginning of the process (Letherby and Bywaters, 2007).

In sum then when researching long term conditions researchers must attend to, reflect and report on all the complex aspects of the research process.

References

Afshar H., 'Muslim women in West Yorkshire: growing up with real and imaginary values amidst conflicting views of self and society', in H. Afshar and M. Maynard (eds), *The Dynamics of 'Race' and Gender: Some Feminist Interventions* (London: Taylor and Francis, 1994).

Afshar H., and M. Maynard (eds), *The Dynamics of 'Race' and Gender: Some Feminist Interventions* (London: Taylor and Francis, 1994).

Blunkett D., *Influence or Irrelevance: Can Social Science Improve Government? Secretary of State's Esrc Lecture Speech 2nd February* (London: Department for Education and Employment, 2000).

Booth T., and W. Booth, 'Sound of silence: narrative research with inarticulate subjects', *Disability and Society*, 11: 1 (1996) 55–69.

Bowling A., *Research Methods in Health*, 2nd edn (Buckingham: Open University Press, 2002).

Brown G., and Harris T., *Social Origins of Depression* (London: Tavistock, 1976).

Bryne-Armstrong H., J. Higgs and D. Horsfall, *Critical Moments in Qualitative Research* (Oxford: Butterworth-Heinemann, 2001).

Burkitt I., 'Social relationships and emotions', *Sociology*, 31: 1(1997) 37–55.

Cannon L.W., E. Higgenbotham and M.L.A. Leung, 'Race and class bias in qualitative research in women', in M.M. Fonnow and J.A. Cook (eds) *Beyond Methodology: Feminist Scholarship as Lived Experience* (Bloomington IN: Indiana University Press, 1991).

Cannon S., 'Social research in stressful settings: difficulties for the sociologist studying the treatment of breast cancer', *Sociology of Health and Illness*, 11: 1 (1989) 62–77.

Colbourne L., 'Split personalities: role conflict between the nurse and the nurse researcher', *Nursing Times Research*, 9: 4 (2004) 297–330.

Collins P., 'Negotiated selves: reflections on "unstructured" interviewing', *Sociological Research Online*, 3: 3 (1998) http://www.socresonline.org.uk/3/3/2.html [last accessed 19 December 2007].

Cotterill P., 'Interviewing women: issues of friendship, vulnerability and power', *Women's Studies International Forum*, 15: 5/6 (1992) 593–606.

Cotterill P., and G. Letherby, 'The Person in the Researcher', in R. Burgess (ed.) *Studies in Qualitative Methodology Volume 4* (London: JAI Press, 1994).

David M., 'Introduction: themed section on evidence-based policy as a concept for modernising governance and social science research', *Social Policy and Society*, 1: 3 (2002) 213–214.

Davis J., N. Watson and S. Cunningham-Burley, 'Learning the lives of disabled children', in P. Christensen and A. James (eds), *Research with Children: Perspectives and Practices* (London: Routledge Falmer, 2000).

Duncombe J., and D. Marsden, '"Stepford Wives" and "Hollow Men"?: doing emotion work, doing gender and "authenticity" in intimate heterosexual relationships', in G. Bendelow and S.J. Williams (eds), *Emotions in Social Life: Critical Themes and Contemporary Issues* (London: Routledge, 1998).

Exley C., and G. Letherby, 'Managing a disrupted lifecourse: issues of identity and emotion work', *Health*, 5: 1 (2001) 112–132.

Fine M., 'Dis-tance and other stances: negotiations of power inside feminist research', in A. Gitlin (ed.), *Power and Method: Political Activism and Educational Research* (London: Routledge, 1994).

Frith H., and C. Kitzinger ' "Emotion work" as a participant resource: a feminist analysis of young women's talk-in-interaction', *Sociology*, 32: 2 (1998) 299–320.

Giddens A., *New Rules of Sociological Method* (London: Macmillan, 1984).

Hallowell N., J. Lawton and S. Gregory, *Reflections on Research: the Realities of Doing Research in the Social Sciences* (Berkshire: Open University Press, 2005).

Hochschild A.R., *The Managed Heart: The Commercialisation of Human Feelings* (London: University of California, 1983).

Hochschild A.R., *The Second Shift* (London: Piakus, 1990).

Hood S., B. Mayall and S. Oliver (eds), *Critical Issues in Social Research* (Buckingham: Open University Press, 1999).

James N. 'Emotional labour: skills and work in the social regulation of feelings', *Sociological Review*, 37: 1 (1989) 5–52.

Jones S.J., 'Reflexivity and feminist practice: ethical dilemmas in negotiating meaning', *Feminism and Psychology* 7: 3 (1997) 348–351.

Kelly L., S. Burton and L. Regan, 'Researching women's lives or studying women's oppression? reflections on what constitutes feminist research', in M. Maynard and J. Purvis (eds), *Researching Women's Lives From a Feminist Perspective* (London: Taylor and Francis, 1994).

Koch T., D. Kralik and D. Sonnack, 'Women living with type II diabetes: the intrusion of illness', *Journal of Clinical Nursing*, 8: 6 (1999) 712–722.

Koch T., and D. Krakik, 'Chronic illness: reflections on a community-based action research programme', *Journal of Advanced Nursing*, 36: 1 (2001) 23–31.

Kralik D., T. Koch and B.M. Brady, 'Pen pals: correspondence as a method for data generation in qualitative research', *Journal of Advanced Nursing*, 31: 4 (2000) 909–917.

Letherby G., 'Challenging dominant discourses: identity and change and the experience of "infertility" and "involuntary childlessness"', *Journal of Gender Studies*, 11: 3 (2002) 277–288.

Letherby G., *Feminist Research in Theory and Practice* (Buckingham: Open University Press, 2003).

Letherby G., and D. Zdrodowski, 'Dear researcher: the use of correspondence as a method within feminist qualitative research', *Gender and Society*, 9: 5 (1995) 576–593.

Letherby G., and P. Bywaters (eds), *Extending Social Research: Application, Implementation and Publication* (Buckingham: Open University Press, 2007).

Lewis V. and M. Kellett, 'Disability', in S. Fraser, V. Lewis, S. Ding, M. Kellett and C. Robinson (eds), *Doing Research with Children and Young People* (London: Sage, 2004).

Locock L. and A. Boaz, 'Research, policy and practice – worlds apart?', *Social Policy and Society*, 3: 4 (2004) 375–384.

Mayall B., S. Hood, and S. Oliver, 'Introduction', in S. Hood, B. Mayall, and S. Oliver (eds), *Critical Issues in Social Research* (Buckingham: Open University Press, 1999).

Miller R.L., and J.D. Brewer, *The A-Z of Social Research: a Dictionary of Key Social Science Research Concepts* (London: Sage, 2003).

Morley L., 'Interrogating patriarchy, the challenges of feminist research', in L. Morley and C. Walsh (eds) *Breaking Boundaries: Women in Higher Education* (London: Taylor and Francis, 1996).

The National Science Foundation, *Workshop on Scientific Foundations of Qualitative Research* (online, 2004) (http://www.nsf.gov/pubs/2004/nsf04219/nsf04219_2.pdf) [last accessed 19 December 2007].

Oakley A., 'Gender, methodology and people's ways of knowing: some problems with feminism and the paradigm debate in social science', *Sociology*, 32: 4 (1998) 707–731.

Oakley A., 'People's ways of knowing: gender and methodology', in S. Hood, B. Mayall and S. Oliver (eds) *Critical Issues in Social Research* (Buckingham: Open University, 1999).

Oakley A., 'Response to "quoting and counting: an autobiographical response to Oakley"', *Sociology*, 38: 1 (2004) 191–192.

Oliver M., 'Emancipatory research: realistic goal or impossible dream', in C. Barnes and G. Mercer (eds) *Doing Disability Research* (Leeds: The Disability Press, 1997).

Packwood A., 'Evidence-based policy; rhetoric and reality', *Social Policy and Society*, 1: 3 (2002) 267–272.

Ramsay K., 'Emotional labour and organisational research: how I learned not to laugh or cry in the field', in S.E. Lyon and J. Busfield (eds), *Methodological Imaginations* (London: Macmillan, 1996).

Reinharz S., *Feminist Methods in Social Research* (Oxford: Oxford University Press, 1992).

Rossiter A., I. Prilleltensky and R. Walsh-Bowers, 'A post modern perspective on modern ethics', in B. Fawcett, B. Featherstone, J. Fook and A. Rossiter (eds) *Practice and Research in Social Work* (London: Routledge, 2000).

Scott A., J. Skea, J. Robinson and E. Shove, *Designing 'Interactive' Environmental Research for Wider Social Relevance*. Special Briefing No. 4 (ESRC Global Environmental Change Programme, 1999).

Sharp K., 'What is Sociology?', in S. Earle and E. Denny (eds), *Sociology for Nurses* (Cambridge: Polity Press, 2005).

Solesbury W., *Evidence Based Policy: Whence It Came and Where It's Going* (London: ESRC Centre for Evidence Based Policy and Practice, Queen Mary, University of London, 2001).

Stacey J., 'Can there be a feminist ethnography?', in S. Gluck and D. Patai (eds), *Women's Words, Women's Words, Women's Words:*

The Feminist Practice of Oral History (New York: Routledge, 1991).

Stalker K., 'Some ethical and methodological issues in research with people with learning difficulties', *Disability and Society*, 13: 1 (1998) 5–19.

Standing K., 'Writing the voices of the less powerful: research on lone mothers', in J. Ribbens and R. Edwards (eds), *Feminist Dilemmas in Qualitative Research* (London: Sage, 1998).

Stanley L., 'Feminist auto/biography and feminist epistemology', in J. Aaron and S. Walby (eds) *Out of the Margins: Women's Studies in the Nineties* (London: Falmer, 1991).

Stanley L., and S. Wise, *Breaking Out Again: Feminist Ontology and Epistemology* (London: Routledge, 1993).

Stanley L., and S. Wise, 'Method, methodology and epistemology in feminist research processes', in L. Stanley (ed.), *Feminist Praxis: Research, Theory and Epistemology* (London: Routledge, 1990).

Strauss A., and J. Corbin, *Basics of Qualitative Research* (London: Sage, 1990).

Stringer E., *Action Research: A Handbook for Practitioners* (Thousand Oaks: Sage, 1996).

Temple B., ' "Collegiate accountability" and bias: the solution to the problem?', *Sociological Research Online*, 2: 4 (1997) http://www.socresonline.org.uk/2/4/8.html [last accessed 19 December 2007].

Truman C., 'Ethics and the ruling relations of research', *Sociological Research Online*, 8: 1 (2003) www.socresonline.org.uk/8/1/truman [last accessed 19 December 2007].

Warren C., *Gender Issues in Field Research* (Newbury Park, CA: Sage, 1988).

Wiles R., S. Heath and G. Crow, *Informed Consent and the Research Process* (Manchester: ESRC Research Methods Programme: Methods Briefing 2, 2005).

Wilkinson S., and C. Kitzinger (eds), *Representing the Other: a Feminism and Psychology Reader* (London: Sage, 1996).

Young E.H., and R. Lee, 'Fieldworker feelings as data: "emotion work" and "feeling rules" in first person accounts of sociological fieldwork', in V. James and J. Gabe (eds), *Health and the Sociology of Emotions* (London: Blackwell, 1996).

II Introduction

Elaine Denny and Sarah Earle

Part I examined some of the theoretical and conceptual approaches to understanding long term conditions within the sociology of health and illness. This part of the book also examined issues around policy and practice, as well as exploring some of the sociological challenges of carrying out research with people living with long term conditions. Part II continues to draw on sociological perspectives; it turns attention to some of the long term conditions that are most prevalent in contemporary society today, and explores the way in the sociological imagination can contribute to nursing practice.

Part II begins with a chapter on Chronic Obstructive Pulmonary Disease (COPD) written by Tom Heller. Formerly known as a spectrum of conditions which included chronic bronchitis, asthmatic bronchitis and emphysema, COPD now persistently features in the list of serious long term conditions, but he asks, 'In whose interest is it that a "new" disease has been created?' In particular, Heller critically examines the role of the multi-national pharmaceutical industry, pointing out that it has found a unique opportunity to market medicines for a condition that will need long term treatment but for which such medicines remain largely ineffective. Heller also examines the social distribution of COPD across the world and argues that there are both social and gendered patterns that provide some clues as to the nature of this largely marginalized disease and the way that people living with COPD can be stigmatized. The author concludes this chapter by focusing on the role of nurses and, in particular, the role of the respiratory nurse specialist in meeting the needs of people living with COPD.

Following on from this, Chapter 5 – written by Lesley Lockyer – focuses on Coronary Heart Disease (CHD), which has now become one of the leading causes of morbidity and mortality in both developed, and many developing, countries. In this chapter Lockyer draws on the model of biographical disruption to explore the differences between professional and lay perceptions of CHD. She notes that given some of the acute and life-threatening symptoms associated with CHD, lay people do not always understand this condition as a long term one. Lockyer also discusses sociological discourses around the relationship of CHD with socio-economic status, lifestyle, and gender differences, arguing that treatment for CHD – such as cardiac rehabilitation programmes – often do not meet the needs of a heterogeneous patient population and, in particular, the needs of women and people from minority ethnic groups. Lockyer suggests that nurses working in primary care, cardiac rehabilitation and acute cardiac care should recognize that whilst they are working within a health care system that purports to offer gender-neutral treatment, this is often far from the case!

In Chapter 6, Cathy E. Lloyd and T. Chas Skinner turn their attention to the subject of diabetes focusing, especially, on issues of policy and practice. Diabetes has become one of the major health concerns of the twenty-first Century, with the incidence and prevalence of this condition increasing rapidly. In this chapter Lloyd and Skinner examine current policy and practice in diabetes care and the implementation of the National Service Framework for diabetes. They also explore different strategies for care, including empowerment and partnership approaches that rely heavily on self-care and which challenge a more traditional, biomedical approach. However, Lloyd and Skinner argue that there are many factors which influence the success of any strategy that relies on self-care. Drawing on empirical research, this chapter concludes by focusing on the issue of (mis)communication between patients and professionals. Lloyd and Skinner argue that nurses and other health professionals should be aware of the way in which miscommunication can threaten patient concordance and, thus, limit the success of any approach that relies on self-care in patients living with diabetes.

The next chapter, which has been written by Jonathon Tritter, focuses on research into patients' understandings and perceptions of living with cancer. Tritter argues that – whether directly or indirectly – the impact of cancer on all of our lives is great. He estimates that up to 30 per cent of people in the developed world will clinically present with cancer at some time in their lives and that although this would have once been seen as a 'death sentence', cancer is no longer perceived in this way. However, he does argue that a central issue for all people with cancer is the sense of suddenly only having a limited time. In his conclusion, Tritter argues that nurses and specialist cancer nurses in particular, have an increasingly important role to play in mediating the care received by people with cancer and their families.

Chapter 8 – by Erica Richardson – explores the experiences of people living with HIV/AIDS (PLWHA). Unlike the other long term conditions discussed within this book, HIV is a communicable disease which is predominantly sexually transmitted and, as such, PLWHA are often feared and highly stigmatized. Richardson begins her chapter by exploring developments in treatment options for PLWHA and current service provision. Next, drawing on research studies on HIV/AIDS carried out in the UK and elsewhere, she focuses on how and why this long term condition became so highly stigmatized. Unlike other work in this area, Richardson's chapter focuses specifically on the lived experiences of PLWHA, rather than on epidemiological or clinical issues. To conclude, Richardson argues that nurses are very well placed to support PLWHA since they are most often their first point of contact within the health service. However, she argues that it is important to understand the fuller complexity of different people's needs in relation to their HIV-positive status in order to support PLWHA effectively.

In Chapter 9, Pauline Savy examines the issue of dementia and the challenges that this condition poses both for the people who have dementia, as well as those who care for them. Savy explores the concept of 'selfhood' and the problem that people with dementia have in articulating selfhood and speaking coherently for themselves. The chapter carefully sets out the discourses of selfhood in dementia and the ways that these shape the obligations of nurses, and other health care practitioners. By focusing on the concept of 'existential labour', Savy argues that this provides a language to describe the experiences of people living with dementia and the possibilities (and limits) for articulating selfhood in the context of dementia.

Chapter 10, which has been written by Ann Mitchell, Elaine Denny and Sarah Earle, focuses on mental health and, specifically, explores social perspectives on depression. This chapter begins by focusing on the fact that depression is thought to be more common than many other physical long term conditions and yet it can still remain ignored or untreated. Mitchell and colleagues examine some of the most dominant contemporary explanations for depression, offering sociological critiques of the biomedical approach to assessment, diagnosis and treatment. The authors present sociological approaches to understanding depression, explaining how these range from those which highlight the role of poverty and disadvantage as a cause of depression, to those which focus critically on the social construction of depression as a disease category. This chapter also examines the role of nurses in mental health work within the context of an ever-changing health service.

Chapter 11, by Sarah Earle, focuses on the issue of obesity and overweight and asks the question: 'Is obesity a long term condition'? The chapter begins with an exploration of how fatness has come to be defined as both a medical and a social problem. It explores confusion and disagreement over the classification of obesity and problems with the anthropological measurement of obesity and overweight in individuals and populations. In spite of this confusion, obesity is widely reported as posing one of the biggest unmet public health needs of the contemporary world. Drawing on some of the theoretical and conceptual frameworks within feminist sociology, disability studies and the sociology of the body, Earle outlines the way in which obesity and overweight are understood within a moral, as well as a medical discourse, in which everyone – everywhere – is at risk. The author also argues that nurses are in a pivotal position to ensure that people who are obese or overweight receive appropriate treatment within a health service, which buys into the notion of an obesity pandemic, but does not provide the resources to enable health care practitioners to provide appropriate and timely services. Drawing on empirical research, Earle also suggests that nurses might want to reflect on their own personal beliefs and behaviour on obesity and question how these might influence patient care.

Finally, the last chapter in this book, written by Elaine Denny, examines the issue of 'heartsink' patients. In this chapter, the author focuses on the intractable conditions of chronic back pain, endometriosis and irritable bowel syndrome to highlight how these conditions are characterized by the fact that: there are problems surrounding diagnosis and treatment of symptoms; they are not of interest to the medical profession; and, their symptoms are often widespread in milder form in the general population. The concept of 'heartsink' refers, quite literally, to the feelings of health professionals on seeing these patients when – usually – little more can be done to improve their symptoms. Drawing and building on the work of other sociologists, Denny concludes the chapter by focusing on what nurses can do to ensure that an understanding of long term conditions such as chronic back pain, endometriosis and irritable bowel syndrome acknowledges the meaning and impact of such conditions on the daily lives of people who suffer from them.

4 'It takes your breath away': the social setting of COPD

Tom Heller

The 'new disease' called COPD

Where has Chronic Obstructive Pulmonary Disease (COPD) sprung from? When I was studying medicine in the 1960s, it didn't feature in our teaching syllabus and yet now it has become a persistent feature in the list of most serious chronic medical conditions. How has this happened, and in whose interest is it that a 'new disease' has been created?

The term COPD has comparatively recently become established shorthand throughout the healthcare fraternity and has become widely used by people labelled with this condition. The term has almost entirely replaced the clinical labels previously used for a spectrum of conditions including chronic bronchitis, asthmatic bronchitis and emphysema. Before 1966 the condition was known in British medical literature and clinical practice as chronic bronchitis, while American physicians tended to use the term emphysema (Petty, 2002). The dispute over nomenclature between the American chest specialists, represented by Benjamin Burrows, and the British camp, championed by the distinguished physician Charles Fletcher, were reconciled when a series of studies failed to find any material difference between the two conditions that happened to have different names on either side of the Atlantic. The term COPD was probably first used at the Aspen Emphysema Conference in 1966 and the unifying hypothesis establishing the common features that inexorably linked the two terms was published soon afterwards in the *Lancet* (Burrows et al., 1966).

Although the term COPD has now become almost universally accepted, for some physicians the change to a unifying term was hard to swallow:

> As a medical student in London in the late 1970s, I was taught that 'COPD' was a very poor term used by Americans to describe three separate diseases – chronic bronchitis, emphysema and asthma. My pedantic teachers emphasized that whilst there was considerable overlap between these conditions, an effort should be made to distinguish between them. Thus I was taught that a patient might present with the symptoms and signs of 'chronic airflow obstruction' or 'chronic airflow limitation' and it was the physician's job to make a diagnosis. Obviously, times have changed! (Bihari, 2003, p. 1046)

More recently, any controversy regarding the naming of the condition has subsided and COPD has been furnished with a straightforward 'working definition' which is widely accepted: 'Chronic obstructive pulmonary disease (COPD) is characterised by airflow obstruction. The airflow obstruction is usually progressive, not fully reversible and does not change markedly over several months. The disease is predominantly caused by smoking' (National Institute for Clinical Excellence [NICE], 2004, p. 2).

Although there has been a considerable degree of consensus about the broad definition of COPD, there remain certain differences in the precise way that it is defined, measured and confirmed in different countries around the world. Notwithstanding these differences, Devereux (2006) reports on studies estimating that approximately 900,000 people are currently recognized as having COPD in England and Wales and that a further 600,000 people in these countries probably have the condition, although they have not yet been diagnosed or labelled (Buist, 2006).

Not only is there an enormous toll of COPD throughout the world (estimated at 600 million people), the condition is one of the few major chronic diseases which is still increasing in incidence (Mathers and Loncar, 2006). By the year 2020 COPD is predicted to become the third leading cause of death worldwide, exceeded only by heart disease and stroke (Murray and Lopez, 1997). The reason for this projected growth in numbers of people with COPD is almost entirely the consequence of current smoking habits of people throughout the world. International COPD statistics reveal that future growth in numbers of people with this condition will come from developing countries and amongst women who, all over the globe, have comparatively recently increased their tobacco consumption.

The social distribution of COPD

COPD is not distributed equally throughout society and there are social and gendered patterns that provide clues to the nature of the disease and the way that it is perceived. COPD is the cause of a considerable health and economic burden in industrialized countries as well as within almost all 'developing' countries. A complex picture is emerging of the patterns of this condition throughout the world.

In the developing world the prevalence of, and mortality from, COPD is still increasing in both sexes (Anto et al., 2001). This increase is bound to continue to occur because the future rise in chronic chest conditions is caused by current increases in tobacco consumption as well as increased industrialization, occupational exposure to particulate matter and air pollution of various types. As well as increases in the disease that relate to comparatively new types of hazardous exposure it appears that some more traditional lifestyles also create additional risk factors for lung damage. One feature that has been quite extensively researched (Chapman et al., 2005) is the particulate damage caused to the lungs of people exposed to stoves within the household that do not have proper ventilation through a chimney. This form of cooking using coal or biomass such as dung or wood is common throughout the developing world and the resultant indoor smoke accounts for 1.6 million deaths worldwide each year. Exposure is highest among women and young children who tend to be inside the house more than men and older children. The good news is that with the installation of decent ventilation systems, such as a chimney to take the smoke to the outside, mortality and morbidity can be considerably reduced (Chapman et al., 2005). The bad news is that many families living in poverty are simply too poor to be able to afford to make the necessary changes to their living conditions.

In the United Kingdom, trends in death rates from COPD are changing rapidly (Pride and Soriano, 2002); the death rate for men is falling, while that for women has been rising over the last 30 years to reflect the changing smoking patterns over this period of time. The socio-economic gradient in COPD is as great, if not greater, than in any other disease (Prescott and Vestbo, 1999). This is caused by the higher incidence of tobacco use amongst people lower down the social class gradient, but also increased exposure to other risk factors such as air and occupational pollutants (Meldrum et al., 2005; Trupin et al., 2003) and the increased incidence of childhood chest infections (Box 4.1).

Box 4.1 Possible causes of the socio-economic gradient in COPD

Low birth weight
Respiratory infections during infancy
Poor housing conditions
Increased house dust mites
Household overcrowding
Home dampness
Community air pollution
Smoking
Passive smoking
Level of education
Occupational dust exposure
Heavy alcohol consumption.

Source: Adapted from Prescott and Vestbo, 1999.

Does working in a dusty environment cause COPD?

Although it might appear self-evident that working in adverse conditions and inhaling 'Dusts, Gases, Vapours or Fumes' (DGVFs) obviously causes lung damage the proof that this is the case has been hard to establish. The mechanisms through which occupational exposure might cause lung damage are not hard to imagine and are entirely similar to the way that cigarette smoke adversely affects lung structure and function over a long period of time, often irreversibly. However for individuals, or indeed whole populations of workers, who have been exposed to DGVFs finding proof of adverse long term effects has been beset with technical and political problems. For a start, the people responsible for creating adverse conditions at the place of work (factory owners and employers), will always attempt to minimize the dangers and act in ways that avoid their liability. Keeping places of work free of dust and other inhaled hazards is potentially technically difficult and may be expensive. The threat of litigation or compensation claims from a damaged workforce will be a strong motivating factor, when factory owners attempt to minimize the scale of resultant health problems or when trying to pin the blame elsewhere. Individual workers and groups of exposed employees or their unions will be on the other side of the politicized argument and seek ways of ensuring a satisfactory working environment and ultimately seeking compensation for any damage that has been caused. Objective epidemiological evidence hasn't been easy to obtain either. Often people working in occupations involving potentially hazardous exposures will have also been exposed to other factors such as tobacco smoke. The development of COPD takes many years during which time each individual worker may have worked in a number of different industries. However, hard evidence has now established links between a large number of occupations and an increased prevalence of COPD. Meldrum et al. (2005) list the occupations positively linked to COPD including: construction, leather, rubber, plastics manufacturing, textiles, food products, spray painters and welders. Certain specific substances have also been shown to cause COPD including: quartz, welding fumes, wood dust, asbestos and solvents.

Different patterns of occupational exposure in the past have created changing patterns of lung-related illness (particularly COPD) amongst the workforce. For example workers in the textile industry develop particular types of lung damage caused by organic contamination of cotton as it is being transformed into garments (Beckett et al., 1994). But more modern industries will also produce their own lung damage (Kreiss, 2007) and the pattern of lung damage from new and 'modern' chemical exposures and contaminants will continue to change and present challenges to individuals and organizations concerned to maintain the health of working people.

Gender differences in the experience of COPD

Several commentators have reviewed the gender-related differences in the development of COPD (Chapman, 2004; Varkey, 2004). They conclude that there are several ways that women seem to be more pre-disposed to the earlier development of COPD. Even given a similar amount of exposure to tobacco smoke they develop COPD at an earlier age and with a greater impairment of lung function than their male counterparts. Chapman (2004) considers that women's airways appear to be more damaged by external stimuli because of differences in lung size and geometry as well as possible hormonal and immunological factors. There does also seem to be a tendency for the disease to be overlooked in women until a greater degree of damage has been sustained: '... there seems a preponderance of women who are affected by early-onset and non-smoking related COPD. Women with COPD also seem to be under-diagnosed by physicians and may have different responses to medical treatment, smoking cessation interventions, and pulmonary rehabilitation programs' (Varkey, 2004, p. 98).

Living with COPD

Are people with COPD met with attitudes and behaviour from other people in society that marks them out as blemished, disgraced or tainted in some way? Is the disease more problematic for people with COPD than for those with similar physical challenges from symptoms caused, for example, by asthma or even lung cancer? Erving Goffman (1963) developed the concept of stigma for people who are seen as different because of an illness (see Chapter 1 for a discussion of Goffman's work on stigma). His work highlighted the fact that particular conditions may create problematic relationships for 'sufferers' with those around them. Some medical conditions may be perceived to label the 'sufferer' as deviant in some way and create a feeling of marginality from 'normal' members of society. Certain medical conditions seem to fall easily into this category, for example people with AIDS or leprosy might find it hard not to be stigmatized by those around them, but is the same true for COPD? The disease differentially affects people in dusty low paid manual jobs, and those who might be seen to have brought the condition on themselves by smoking. In addition, the medical profession may give the condition low priority because there are no dramatic or technologically sophisticated interventions to offer patients, and available treatments have limited effectiveness.

Certainly, a proportion of people with COPD feel themselves to be both stigmatized and stereotyped. A survey of 649 people with COPD (Emphysema.net 2005) found that almost 90 per cent believed that others thought they had brought on their lung condition themselves. Other surveys of people with COPD have found that psychosocially related variables such as feelings of social and emotional isolation have a stronger influence of peoples' quality of life than even biomedical variables such as shortness of breath (Fraser et al., 2006). People who smoke are increasingly being stigmatized and socially isolated because of their habit. Although some commentators relish this change in social marginalization (Bayer and Stuber, 2006), it does seem rather harsh to stigmatize those people who are now victims of a disease induced by the socially accepted habits of a previous era:

> In the last half century the cigarette has been transformed. The fragrant has become foul. ... An emblem of attraction has become repulsive. A mark of sociability has become deviant. A public behaviour is now virtually private. Not only has the meaning of the cigarette been transformed but even more the meaning of the smoker [who] has become a pariah ... the object of scorn and hostility. (Bayer and Stuber, 2006, p. 47)

The realities of daily living with COPD as a disabling, limiting condition have been studied by a number of researchers. Odencrants, Ehnfors and Grobe (2005) considered the experiences of people with COPD and their relationship to food. Many reported significant problems associated with shopping, cooking and eating a meal. Three of their research subjects described difficult experiences relating to food, for example:

> tired, very tired. I cannot manage standing there peeling an onion. It's not like me at all.

...then I do not succeed, so I feel like a failure; I've been standing there making food and then I can't eat it up.

Oh my God I have not eaten anything yet, and I'm already full. (Odencrants, Ehnfors and Grobe 2005, pp. 233–235)

And the repeated effort of shopping, preparing, cooking and eating food regularly becomes an exhausting process that needs to be negotiated several times each day: 'I just sit still an hour after eating, and only then do I start washing the dishes at my own pace' (Odencrants, Ehnfors and Grobe, 2005, p. 235).

Guthrie, Hill and Muers (2001) looked at the entire experience of people living with COPD in Leeds and reported the fear and restrictions that continual breathlessness can bring about. Their respondents planned their lives in order to avoid strenuous activity: '...many of our patients' lives were shadowed by fear. External threats often formed a foundation for anxiety of almost overwhelming magnitude when added to the daily struggle to get one's breath and perform daily duties in spite of physical constraints' (Guthrie, Hill and Muers, 2001, p. 200).

The social isolation associated with COPD has often been commented on by researchers in this field. Barnett (2005) reported the frustration that follows the loss of social activity experienced by many people with COPD who may need to preserve their energy simply in order to get through each day. In turn, exhaustion and breathlessness can lead to loss of their role within the family and loss of intimacy in personal relationships. The effort of going out and having fun may become the last thing on someone's list of things to do. Paradoxically it appears that social interaction and community participation are features most valued by people with COPD (Williams et al., 2007).

People with COPD seem to have very low expectations for their own health, for the level of help that they can anticipate and for the way that they might be treated when in contact with the National Health Service (NHS). This is often translated into a passiveness and resignation through the course of their disease during which time they have to, '...put up with so much and demand so very little' (Mussell, 2007). Balancing the need for external help with the very real knowledge for the person with COPD that they alone are experiencing the difficult breathing and have just themselves to draw the next breath has been commented on by Fraser et al. (2006). People with COPD become experts themselves in managing their own breathing and energy levels and can become upset or panic stricken when well meaning people, including carers and family members, try to help:

> They want to help, but ... they have no concept of what I'm going through at all...Finally I said, 'Back off!' because I had to be totally alone to...just concentrate on...stop...breathe...Sometimes it takes a while to get a handle on it...but you gotta do it yourself 'cause nobody else can. (Fraser et al., 2006, p. 553)

When chest infections or other types of exacerbation develop all these fears and feelings worsen for the person with COPD, and it is no surprise that researchers at the more clinical end of the spectrum have found high levels of anxiety and depression and generally low quality of life scores (Cleland et al., 2007; Wagena et al., 2005).

Drug company interest and involvement

For Public Health strategists and frontline clinical workers the rapid growth in the size of the problem of COPD represents an enormous challenge. However, this phenomenon also represents an enormous market for medication, and the multinational pharmaceutical industry has not been slow to appreciate this fact. In many ways, the newly created, unified disease of COPD represents the ideal marketing opportunity: 'Raising awareness of COPD and developing drugs that address this indication represents a major area of unmet medical need and is consequently a major opportunity for drug developers' (Thomson, 2006, p. 1).

Box 4.2   COPD as a marketing opportunity

In researching this part of the chapter, I used a standard search engine to look for items under the term *'COPD marketing opportunities'*. These are some quotations taken from the websites of various marketing organizations. They share the view that COPD has become a highly lucrative market. All were accessed on 9 February 2007. By the time you read this chapter new marketing opportunities in this field will be being offered.

It is estimated that the global annual sales in the asthma and COPD market are due to increase by over $10 billion US dollars within the next five years and then remain flat thereafter. Will you make use of this transforming market & increasing potential before it's too late? http://www.smi-online.co.uk/events/overview.asp?is=4&ref=2508

COPD is a disease that will grow in importance in the future and it will have a major impact on society, particular amongst those that smoke. At the moment, although new treatments are being developed for COPD the pharmaceutical market remains undeveloped. There will be a high demand for effective medicines and so COPD should be an area of interest for pharmaceutical companies who specialise in the respiratory therapeutic field. http://www.pharmiweb.com/Features/feature.asp?ROW_ID=772

New product launches, including Spiriva and roflumilast, combined with an aging population and approval of combination ICS & LABA therapies in COPD, will see the market value of smoker's lung rise to at least $5.5 billion by 2011, with Pfizer emerging as a major player. Given that approximately 50 per cent of the 30 million COPD patients in the seven major markets are undiagnosed, increased awareness coupled with a reduction in lung function deterioration will prove critical to unlocking the true COPD patient potential. http://www.leaddiscovery.co.uk/reports/Combinations%20breathe%20life%20into%20the%20asthma%20and%20COPD%20markets.html

Box 4.2 illustrates some of the ways in which the pharmaceutical industry has identified COPD as a growth area for its attention. It is natural enough and entirely legitimate that companies making appropriate products will want to increase their sales aimed at this attractive and lucrative sector of the market. The COPD market is dominated by seven multinational drug companies who together sold respiratory medication to the value of $41 billion in 2005. This sector of the market is projected to grow to $65 billion by the year 2014 (Thomson, 2006). COPD is especially attractive to the makers of medication because, unlike antibiotics for acute infections, none of the respiratory medication is curative. Once a person with COPD is put on an apparently symptom-relieving medication they will almost certainly remain on it for many years. Box 4.3 shows that inhaled COPD medication is not cheap and individual pharmaceutical companies can expect huge rewards for successfully marketed drugs. Tiotropium (Spiriva®), manufactured by Boehringer Inglelheim, generated sales of 950 million euros (approx. £630 million), in the year 2005, while GlaxoSmithKline plc had another 'blockbuster' with their combination therapy Serevent® generating sales of £3 billion in the same year (Thomson, 2006). It is also interesting to note that the NHS puts few restrictions on prescribing expensive inhaled medication, yet struggles to pay for rehabilitation classes that might help people with COPD and be effective in slowing the rate of decline in pulmonary function.

Box 4.3 Cost of Bronchodilator therapies licensed for use in COPD

Medication	30 day cost (£)
Salbutamol/ipratropium (Combivent) 100mcg/20 mcg	7.74
Formoterol (Oxis) 12 mcg Turbohaler	24.80
Salmeterol (Serevent) 25 mcg Evohaler	31.46
Tiotropium (Spiriva) Handihaler	37.62

Drug companies and involvement in the COPD nexus

It is in the interest of the drug industry to continue to make concerted efforts to influence the networks that determine the way that various diseases are perceived as well as treated. This has been a growing trend in the marketing of medication across all disease sectors. Multinational drug companies use a significant proportion of their resources to make sure that they are 'at the table' when research, education, public awareness and even regulation of medication is being determined.

The world of COPD provides many examples where the reach of drug companies has stretched to include most aspects of the way that this 'new' disease is currently conceptualized and managed. This, in itself, is not necessarily harmful, but it does mean that no decisions about the way that the disease is handled throughout the world will be taken without the interests of the multinational drug industry being considered. The Global Initiative for Chronic Obstructive Lung Disease, usually known as GOLD, was established in 1997. This widely respected organization has brought together many of the world's leading public health bodies such as the National Institutes of Health from the United States and the World Health Organization, 'to raise awareness of COPD and to improve prevention and treatment of this lung disease'. There can be little doubt about the good intentions of this organization and its pronouncements on the way that COPD should be diagnosed, managed and prevented have indeed become the 'GOLD standard'. However even a cursory exploration of the GOLD website http://goldcopd.com/index.asp?l1=1&l2=0 (last accessed in September 2008), demonstrates some of the ways that multinational drug companies ensure that their voice is heard at the highest level within the organization. GOLD's reports and activities are funded by unrestricted educational grants from 14 commercial sponsors including all the major multinational pharmaceutical companies that produce respiratory medication. The members of the various GOLD committees are required to disclose their relationships with profit-making organizations and almost all the GOLD committee members (see Box 4.4), have disclosed significant benefits to themselves or their research departments emanating from drug companies.

Box 4.4 Examples of disclosure statements of GOLD committee members

Executive committee member A:

Personal benefits >$10,000:	Surface therapeutics
Personal benefits >$10,000:	Altana, AstraZeneca, Boehringer Ingelheim, GlaxoSmithKline, Novartis, Pfizer.
Shares:	None.
Non-personal interests >$10,000:	AstraZeneca, Boehringer Ingelheim, GlaxoSmithKline, Mitsubishi, Novartis, Pfizer.

Science committee member B:

Personal benefits <$10,000:	Almirallprodesfarma, Altana, AstraZeneca, GlaxoSmithKline, Novartis, Procter/Gamble, Wonca.
Personal benefits >$10,000:	Boehringer Ingelheim/Pfizer.
Shares <$10,000:	Genetrix, SL.
Non-personal interests <$10,000:	Boehringer Ingelheim/Pfizer, Esteve.

Source: http://goldcopd.com/index.asp?l1=1&l2=0 (last accessed 21 September 2008)

All drug companies are required to carry out research on the drugs that they intend to introduce into the market and most will also continue to sponsor research once the medication is in clinical use. But does research that has been funded by drug companies arrive at different conclusion from similar work conducted by independent organizations? There is growing evidence (Lexchin et al., 2003) that drug company funded research is associated with outcomes that are favourable to those pharmaceutical companies. The bias is not thought to be related to the quality of the research itself, but to the way that drug companies might compare their drugs with inappropriate comparators, and of course their reluctance to publish any findings that are not favourable to their product. Comparing drug company analyzes of the effectiveness of their medication with independent research (in this case independent Cochrane reviews) concluded: 'Industry supported reviews of drugs should be read with caution as they were less transparent, had few reservations about methodological limitations of the included trials, and had more favourable conclusions than the corresponding Cochrane reviews' (Jørgensen et al., 2006, p. 782).

The influence of drug company research is increasing and since 1994 biotechnology and drug companies have provided funding for an increasing proportion of the most influential research papers (Patsopoulos et al., 2006).

The ways that drug companies seek to exert pressure on doctors who may be influenced in their prescribing patterns has been well documented (Abbasi and Smith, 2003). Various campaigns such as the 'No Free Lunch' campaign http://www.nofreelunch.org/reqreading.htm, have been established to counter the advertising and biased promotional activities that are aimed at doctors. However, the relationship between the pharmaceutical industry and patient groups has achieved less prominence (Herxheimer, 2003). Patient groups have been described as conduits, albeit unsuspectingly, for drug companies to promote their products, and as 'ground troops' to be used to lobby governments for increased access to new drugs (Ferner and McDowell, 2006). Although they are supposed to be grassroots organizations, one analyst at least considers that some patient groups 'are perilously close to becoming extensions of pharmaceutical companies' marketing departments'. (Drummond Rennie, Professor of medicine at the University of California, quoted in Marshall and Aldhous, 2006). In the field of COPD there are several active international patient groups sponsored by 'Big Pharma'. For example the International COPD Coalition (http://www.internationalcopd.org/) (last accessed 22 September 2008), is sponsored by Pfizer, Atlanta Pharma, Boehringer Ingelheim, GlaxoSmithKline, AstraZeneca and Novartis. And the European Federation of Allergy and Airways Diseases Patients Associations (EFA) (http://www.efanet.org/) (last accessed 22 September 2008), is sponsored by AstraZeneca, GlaxoSmithKline, Novartis and UCB Pharma. For other patient groups it is difficult to determine the extent of their financial backing. Ball et al. (2006) surveyed 69 significant patient organizations and found it virtually impossible to uncover the financial backing that was being provided by the pharmaceutical companies. GlaxoSmithKline invested £386,000 over two years in the British Lung Foundation's Baby Breathe Easy programme, which supports parents and carers of young children and babies with chest problems.

Treating COPD: what works and what doesn't?

COPD is, by definition, a chronic condition and it probably only becomes apparent and symptomatic after substantial, and probably irreversible lung damage has taken place (Sabroe et al., 2007). Any treatment or relief of symptoms is working against difficult odds and improvement will be virtually impossible if the factors that have caused the condition are not reversed. For example, no treatment for a person with COPD who smokes will be as effective as quitting smoking; removing a person from a dusty, damaging occupation will also slow the progress of the disease.

Demonstrating the effectiveness, or otherwise, of treatments for COPD is notoriously complex and debates continue regarding the effectiveness of almost all medical treatments. Any research in this area will have to recruit a large number of people who will need to be followed for a long period of time and compared with other people with the same amount of lung damage and similar symptoms in order to demonstrate whether the treatment has had any statistically different effect in the different groups. No wonder it is usually only drug companies that can afford to undertake these large clinical trials. One of the most recent drug industry sponsored trials (Calverley et al., 2007), rather flamboyantly and possibly prematurely called TORCH (Towards a Revolution in COPD Health) followed over six thousand people with COPD and 'failed to reach a clinically useful conclusion' (*British Medical Journal* [BMJ], 2007). The trial compared four different treatment regimes but because four out of ten people dropped out of the trial for various reasons the findings were borderline and difficult to interpret. Only one of the treatments improved mortality rates more than the placebo and this difference was not strictly statistically significant. There were some statistically significant benefits from therapy in slowing the rate of decline in lung function.

The study also found unintended outcomes from the use of some of the inhaled medication; for example the incidence of pneumonia was increased in two of the treatment groups when compared with the people using only placebo treatment. Other detailed research studies have thrown doubt on the long term beneficial effects of some of the other common treatments for COPD. Soriano et al. (2007) followed almost four thousand people with COPD who used inhaled steroid therapy. She found that although there was some improvement in lung function for the first six months of treatment, for the next two and a half years of follow up in the study there was no significant difference between the treatment group and those using placebo.

Even if the long term effectiveness of some of the conventional drug-based treatments for COPD are rather disappointing it is important not to become too despondent or nihilistic about the possibility of helping people who are unfortunate enough to develop this condition. Celli (2006) reviewed the evidence for a wide range of approaches and found cause for optimism in a number of non drug-based approaches including smoking cessation and pulmonary rehabilitation. Pulmonary rehabilitation can mean different things in different contexts. Usually it involves a multidisciplinary programme of education and care for people who already have damaged lung function. Although the therapy may take place in group settings it should be individually tailored to optimize each patient's physical and social performance and autonomy (Ries et al., 2007). Pulmonary rehabilitation leads to statistically significant and clinically meaningful improvements in health-related quality of life, functional exercise capacity, and maximum exercise capacity in patients with stable COPD.

Regular physical activity by itself has also been found to be enormously beneficial in the treatment of COPD. In a previous era it may have been suggested to people who have lung damage such as COPD that they should rest, take things easy and not consider pushing their exercise levels. However this approach has now been entirely superseded by various forms of exercise training that provide general conditioning and improves the quality of life for people with COPD. Garcia-Aymerich et al. (2006) followed over 2,300 people with COPD and found that those who continued with a level of activity at least equivalent to a couple of hours of walking or cycling each week had a 30–40 per cent reduction in hospital admission due to COPD and a similar reduction in respiratory mortality.

Nursing people with COPD

Many of the traditional hierarchical structures that for the last two hundred years have governed medicine and the care of people with long term conditions are currently undergoing rapid change. The old certainties in which doctors assumed themselves to be at the top of the pile and ordered nurses what to do are being challenged on many fronts. Of course the nurses themselves are keen to improve their status, continue to develop their own research agenda and challenge many of the previously sacrosanct bastions of doctors' power and authority. Managers of health care systems delight in these realignments and can immediately see the benefits of a service in which many of the roles traditionally assigned to (expensive and usually rigid) doctors can be equally well performed by (comparatively cheap and possibly pliable) nurses.

Nurse practitioners have been found to perform better than doctors in plenty of settings. Many studies in primary care have found that people prefer to see the nurse (Horrocks et al., 2002); They are given longer consultations, sent for more investigations and the quality of care has been judged to be superior to that offered by primary care physicians. At the same time there is an enormous concentration of officially sanctioned effort attempting to keep people, even when seriously ill, out of (expensive again) hospital facilities. In the world of COPD care these forces have come together to create the comparatively new phenomenon of the Respiratory Nurse Specialist (RNS). Rafferty and Elborn (2002) pertinently asked if this new breed of health worker could run a COPD clinic better than physicians. They could find no statistically significant differences in outcomes measuring health status or future hospital admission rates. Although a later review of published evidence (Taylor et al., 2005) found little or no evidence that nurse led chronic disease management innovations were more effective than 'usual care' in people with COPD. the push towards RNS development continues. Managers, again, are delighted that specialist nurse care is cost-effective (Gordois, 2002) and has improved care for people with acute exacerbations of COPD. Under the care of an RNS nurse continuity was improved, fewer people were admitted to hospital and then stayed for shorter periods of time. Other innovations that have proved effective include the creation of 'hospital at home' facilities run by RNS teams providing a service for people who would have otherwise been admitted to hospital with an acute exacerbation (Hernandez et al., 2003).

Although there would seem to be conditions for tension between physicians and nurses over the battleground in relation to who should provide care for people with COPD, in practice there seems to be a remarkable consensus working towards multi-professional teams and various models of 'integrated' care (Fletcher and Hernandez, 2006). There's plenty of work for everyone in the COPD arena:

Nurses have proven themselves to be a well educated, experienced and caring resource to lead respiratory services into the future and this resource will need to continue to grow as the numbers of people

living with respiratory conditions increase. In line with this continuing growth, respiratory nurses need to be more self-critical and educational models should be adapted to society demands. Whatever the
drivers, our time has come! (Fletcher and Hernandez, 2006, p. 178)

Despite advances in the treatment of COPD and the continuing
development of specialist professional roles, it is usually considered
that the condition eventually leads to functional decline, increasing shortness of breath and ultimately death. The symptoms,
such as fighting for breath towards the end of life, are horrid, persistent and frightening for the people with COPD and for their
carers. Two carers describe their observations following the death
of the people they have cared for (Elkington et al., 2004): "'She
had panic attacks terrible didn't she, where she'd wake up and
she couldn't breathe even with the oxygen". "I would say there
was a tremendous mixture in him of finding the whole business
absolutely intolerable and horrendous and at the same time being
very afraid of death"' (Elkington et al., 2004, p. 442).

Several commentators have compared the final stages of
COPD with the terminal phases of lung cancer (Goodridge,
2007; Gore et al., 2000). The comparison usually comes out
favourably for people with lung cancer who appear to get better
palliative care and whose suffering seems well acknowledged
and dealt with by health professionals. People with COPD
continue to have a particularly hard time in the last years of
their life and specialist palliative care services, such as hospice
care, are often denied to them. More people with COPD die
in hospital than people with lung cancer. They have similar
degrees of pain, shortness of breath, sickness, anxiety, depression and other distressing and degrading symptoms yet fewer
opportunities for symptom control or supportive therapies. In
particular the evidence base regarding adequate management
of shortness of breath lags far behind that for pain management (Goodridge, 2007). Perhaps these findings highlight the
lack of progress towards de-stigmatizing COPD.

Summary

Studying the phenomenon of COPD has given us the opportunity to consider some of the social and sociological
facets surrounding the care of people with long term medical

conditions. COPD is not scattered at random throughout society, but demonstrates very strong, socially determined patterns. This is a problematic condition that targets socially disadvantaged people and those living in poverty throughout the world. Health care professionals, doctors and nurses, have a mixed relationship with this condition and in many respects it continues to remain stigmatized and starved of proper attention. On the other hand the multinational drug industry has focussed its considerable resources on this condition. Always with an eye to marketing opportunities they perceive a chronic condition in which people need long term treatment and symptom relief that may be expensive yet remains only marginally effective. People with this condition live a long time using large quantities of medication of variable effectiveness. Non drug-based interventions that are of proven effectiveness, such as respiratory rehabilitation and exercise regimes, are starved of funds and lack widespread deployment. It is hard to avoid the conclusion that the lack of resources for simple rehabilitation measures has come about because so much money has been spent on medication. And at the end of life, after possibly many years of increasingly problematic symptoms and frequent hospital admissions, people with COPD may not receive the degree of palliative and ultimately terminal care afforded to others who happen to have conditions that have fought off stigma and attracted advocates and detailed attention.

References

Abbasi K., and R. Smith, 'No more free lunches', *British Medical Journal*, 326 (2003) 1155–1156.

Anto J., P. Vermeire, J. Vestbo and J. Sunyer, 'Epidemiology of chronic obstructive pulmonary disease', *European Respiratory Journal*, 17 (2001) 982–984.

Ball D., K. Tisocki and A. Herxheimer, 'Advertising and disclosure of funding on patient organisation websites: a cross-sectional survey', *BMC Public Health* (2006) http://www.biomedcentral.com/content/pdf/1471-2458-6-201.pdf (last accessed 20 April 2007).

Barnett M., 'Chronic obstructive pulmonary disease: a phenomenological study of patients' experiences', *Journal of Clinical Nursing*, 14 (2005) 805–812.

Bayer R., and J. Stuber, 'Tobacco control, stigma and public health: rethinking the relations', *American Journal of Public Health*, 46 (2006) 47–50.

Beckett W., C. Pope, X. Xu and D. Christiani, 'Women's respiratory health in the cotton textile industry: an analysis of respiratory symptoms in 973 non-smoking female workers', *Occupational and Environmental Medicine*, 51 (1994) 14–18.

Bihari D., 'The Americanisation of British medicine – COPD or CAO/CAL?' Rapid response to D. Price, and M. Duerden (2003) 'Chronic obstructive pulmonary disease' *British Medical Journal*, 326 (2003) 1046–1047. http://www.bmj.com/cgi/eletters/326/7398/1046#32296 (last accessed 9 February 2007).

British Medical Journal (BMJ) News, 'Treatments for COPD may not prolong survival', 334 (2007) 448.

Buist S., 'COPD: a common disease that is preventable and treatable', *Primary Care Respiratory Journal*, 15 (2006) 7–9.

Burrows B., C. Fletcher and B. Heard, 'The emphysematous and bronchial types of chronic airway obstruction: a clinopathological study of patients in London and Chicago', *Lancet*, 1 (1966) 830–835.

Calverley P., J. Anderson, B. Celli, G. Ferguson, C. Jenkins, P. Jones, J. Yates and J. Vestbo, 'Salmeterol and fluticasone propionate and survival in chronic obstructive pulmonary disease', *New England Journal of Medicine*, 356 (2007) 775–789.

Celli B., 'Chronic obstructive pulmonary disease: from unjustified nihilism to evidence-based optimism', *Proceedings of the American Thoracic Society*, 3 (2006) 58–65.

Chapman K., 'Chronic obstructive pulmonary disease: are women more susceptible than men?', *Clinics in Chest Medicine*, 25 (2004) 331–341.

Chapman R., H. Xingzhou, A. Blair and L. Qing, 'Improvement in household stoves and risk of chronic onstructive pulmonary disease in Xuanwei, China: retrospective cohort study', *British Medical Journal*, 331 (2005) 1050–1056.

Cleland J., A. Lee and S. Hall, 'Associations of depression and anxiety with gender, age, health-related quality of life and symptoms in primary care COPD patients', *Family Practice*, 24 (2007) 217–223.

Devereux G., 'Definition, epidemiology and risk factors: ABC of chronic obstructive pulmonary disease', *British Medical Journal*, 332 (2006) 1142–1144.

Elkington H., P. White, J. Addington-Hall, R. Higgs and C. Pettinari, 'The last year of life of COPD: a qualitative study of symptoms and services', *Respiratory Medicine*, 98 (2004) 439–445.

Emphysema.net, 'COPD: challenging symptoms, stigma and stereotypes', Patient survey fact sheet (2005) www.emphysema.net/Survey_Fact_Sheet.htm (last accessed 4 May 2007).

Ferner R., and S. McDowell, 'How NICE may be outflanked', *British Medical Journal*, 332 (2006) 1268–1271.

Fletcher M., and C. Hernandez, 'An exciting future for respiratory nurses?', *Chronic Respiratory Disease*, 3 (2006) 177–178.

Fraser D., C. Kee and P. Minik, 'Living with chronic obstructive pulmonary disease: insiders' perspectives', *Journal of Advanced Nursing*, 55 (2006) 550–558.

Garcia-Aymerich J., P. Lange, M. Benet, P. Schnohr and J. Anto, 'Regular physical activity reduces hospital admission and mortality in chronic obstructive pulmonary disease: a population based cohort study', *Thorax*, 61 (2006) 772–778.

Goffman E., *Stigma: Notes on the Management of Spoiled Identity* (New York: Simon and Schuster, 1963).

Goodridge D., 'COPD as a life-limiting illness: implications for advanced practice nurses', *Topics in Advanced Practice Nursing e-Journal*, 6 (2007) 4.

Gordois A., 'The cost-effectiveness of outreach respiratory care for COPD patients', *Professional Nurse*, 17 (2002) 504.

Gore J., C. Brophy and M. Greenstone, 'How well do we care for patients with end stage chronic obstructive pulmonary disease (COPD)? A comparison of palliative care and quality of life in COPD and lung cancer', *Thorax*, 55 (2000) 1000–1006.

Guthrie S., K. Hill and M. Muers, 'Living with severe COPD. A qualitative exploration of the experience of patients in Leeds', *Respiratory Medicine*, 95 (2001) 196–204.

Hernandez C., C. Casas, and J. Escarrabill, 'Home hospitalisation of exacerbated chronic obstructive pulmonary disease patients', *European Respiratory Journal*, 21 (2003) 58–67.

Herxheimer A., 'Relationships between the pharmaceutical industry and patients' organisations', *British Medical Journal*, 326 (2003) 1208–1210.

Horrocks S., E. Anderson and C. Salisbury, 'Systematic review of whether nurse practitioners working in primary care can provide equivalent care to doctors', *British Medical Journal*, 324 (2002) 819–823.

Jørgensen A., J. Hilden and P. Gøtzsche, 'Cochrane reviews compared with industry supported meta-analyses and other meta-analyses of the same drugs: systematic review', *British Medical Journal*, 333 (2006) 782–787.

Kreiss K., 'Emerging opportunities to prevent occupational lung disease' *Occupational and Environmental Medicine*, 64 (2007) 499–500.

Lexchin J., L. Bero, B. Djulbegovic and O. Clark, 'Pharmaceutical industry sponsorship and research outcome and quality: systematic review', *British Medical Journal*, 326 (2003) 1167–1170.

Marshall J., and R. Aldhous, 'Patient groups special: swallowing the best advice?', *New Scientist*, 2575 (2006) 18–22.

Mathers C., and D. Loncar, 'Projections of Global Mortality and Burden of Disease from 2002 to 2030' *PLoS Medicine*, 3 (11) (2006) e442 doi:10.1371/journal.pmed.0030442 http://medicine.plosjournals. org/perlserv/?request=get-document&doi=10.1371%2Fjournal. pmed.0030442 (last accessed 9 February 2007).

Meldrum M., R. Rawbone, A. Curran and D Fishwick, 'The role of occupation in the development of chronic obstructive pulmonary disease (COPD)', *Occupational and Environmental Medicine*, 62 (2005) 212–214.

Murray C., and A. Lopez, 'Alternative projections of mortality and disability by cause 1990–2020: Global Burden of Disease Study', *Lancet*, 349 (1997) 1498–1504.

Mussell L., *Personal communication* (October 2007).

National Institute for Clinical Excellence (NICE), 'Chronic obstructive pulmonary disease: Management of chronic obstructive disease in adults in primary and secondary care', *Clinical Guideline 12* (London: NICE, 2004). http://www.nice.org.uk/pdf/ CG012quickrefguide.pdf (last accessed 9 January 2007)

Odencrants S., M. Ehnfors and S. Grobe, 'Living with chronic obstructive pulmonary disease: Part 1. Struggling with meal-related situations: experiences among persons with COPD', *Scandinavian Journal of Caring Sciences*, 19 (2005) 230–239.

Patsopoulos N., J. Ioannidis and A. Analatos, 'Origin and funding of the most frequently cited papers in medicine: database analysis', *British Medical Journal*, 332 (2006) 1062–1064.

Petty T., 'COPD in perspective', *Chest*, 121 (2002) 116S–120S.

Prescott E., and J. Vestbo, 'Socioeconomic status and chronic obstructive pulmonary disease', *Thorax*, 54 (1999) 737–741.

Pride N., and J. Soriano, 'Chronic obstructive pulmonary disease in the United Kingdom: trends in mortality, morbidity and smoking', *Current Opinion in Pulmonary Medicine*, 8 (2002) 95–101.

Rafferty S., and J. Elborn, 'Do nurses do it better? Can nurse led clinics produce outcomes in respiratory care that are as effective as those produced by respiratory physicians', *Thorax*, 57 (2002) 659–660.

Ries A., G. Bauldoff, B. Carlin, R. Casaburi, C. Emery, D. Mahler, B. Make, C. Rochester, R. ZuWallack and C. Herrerias, 'Pulmonary rehabilitation executive summary', *Chest*, 131 (2007) S1–S3.

Sabroe I., L. Parker, P. Calverley, S. Dower and M. Whyte, 'Pathological networking: a new approach to understanding COPD', *Thorax*, 62 (2007) 733–738.

Sin. Soriano J. et al., 'A pooled analysis of FEV1 decline in COPD patients randomized to inhaled corticosteroids or placebo', *Chest*, 131 (2007) 682–689.

Taylor S., B. Candy, R. Bryar, J. Ramsay, H. Vrijhoef, G. Esmond, J. Wedzicha and C. Griffiths, 'Effectiveness of innovations in nurse led chronic disease management for patients with chronic obstructive pulmonary disease: systematic review of evidence', *British Medical Journal*, 331 (2005) 485–492.

Thomson C., *COPD Drug Discovery: How New Generation Therapies Seek to Target Underlying Disease* (Dublin: Drug and Market Development Publishing, 2006).

Trupin L., G. Earnest, M. San Pedro, J. Balmes, M. Eisner, E. Yelin, P. Katz and P. Blanc, 'The occupational burden of chronic obstructive pulmonary disease', *European Respiratory Journal*, 22 (2003) 462–469.

Varkey A., 'Chronic obstructive pulmonary disease in women; exploring gender differences', *Current Opinion in Pulmonary Medicine*, 10 (2004) 98–103.

Wagena E., W. Arrindell, E. Wouters and C. Schayck, 'Are patients with COPD psychologically distressed?', *European Respiratory Journal*, 26 (2005) 242–248.

Williams V., A. Bruton, C. Ellis-Hill and K. McPherson, 'What really matters to patients living with chronic obstructive pulmonary disease? An exploratory study', *Chronic Respiratory Disease*, 4 (2007) 77–85.

5 Coronary heart disease: moving from acute to long-term accounts

Lesley Lockyer

Introduction

Coronary Heart Disease (CHD) has been classified since Heberden in 1768 first described Angina Pectoris, but more recent history has witnessed the development of theories about the relationship between diet, lifestyle, personality and CHD. Sociologists and other social scientists have also highlighted the social nature of CHD and the implications of this for practice. Professional accounts portray the middle aged white male as a 'gold standard' typical of the type of person who gets CHD. Consequently, the developed standardized care may not be appropriate for women, older people and people from other ethnic backgrounds.

The chapter begins by outlining the nature of the CHD pandemic, exploring how and why perceptions and ideas about CHD have changed over time. Following this, the chapter explores both professional and lay accounts of CHD, examining the gendered experiences of this long-term condition. It concludes by drawing together this discussion, and using Bury's (1991) model of biographical disruption presents a conceptual model of CHD as a chronic degenerative illness, discussing the implications of this for nurses.

Morbidity and mortality associated with coronary heart disease

Interest in CHD by natural and social scientists has been fuelled by the sheer numbers of men and women who develop this long-term condition. Not only is it a major health and social problem in the United Kingdom and other similarly developed countries where cardiovascular diseases are the main cause of death and one of the main causes of premature death and chronic illness (Allender et al., 2006), but also in the developing world. For example, the World Health Organization estimates that countries in South east Asia will have CHD as their major cause of morbidity and mortality within the next couple of decades; this disease is now described as a pandemic (Mackay and Mensah, 2004).

Death rates due to CHD in the United Kingdom have fallen since the 1970s. However this fall has been greatest among the higher socio-economic groups, widening the social class gradients in CHD mortality and morbidity. In 1997 it was estimated that 5,000 lives are lost each year from CHD through the premature mortality of men aged 20 to 64 due to social class differences; this is reflected in the prevalence of CHD morbidity which is more common in those in lower socio-economic groups (Allender et al., 2006). The level of mortality among women in the United Kingdom from CHD is lower than in men however women's levels are declining at a slower rate than men's (Sharp, 1994). In 2004 a total of 105,842 men and women died from CHD, 11,396 men and 2,848 women were aged less than 65 years when they died (Allender et al., 2006).

Morbidity data are much more difficult than mortality data to collect as not all affected individuals seek medical assistance and, even when they do, symptoms may not be correctly diagnosed nor is there a single database where morbidity data are collated. The prevalence of CHD as a long-term condition can

Table 5.1 Estimated prevalence of CHD morbidity in the United Kingdom

	Men (All ages)	Women (All ages)
Myocardial infarction	870,000	419,000
Angina	> 1 million	> 840,000
Heart failure	506,000	406,000

Source: Adapted from Allender et al., 2006.

be assessed through statistics detailing the numbers of men and women living who have had a Myocardial Infarction (MI), suffer with angina or who live with heart failure. The British Heart Foundation statistics database publish figures year on year (Table 5.1) which give an indication of aspects of CHD morbidity.

Historical accounts of coronary heart disease: developing the gendered discourse

New centuries and new situations within the UK public health arena have swept away the old communicable diseases such as cholera and typhoid as the main causes of morbidity and mortality and replaced them with new communicable diseases such as HIV and AIDS (see Chapter 8) and non communicable diseases such as cancer (see Chapter 7) and CHD. However, it is fair to suggest that CHD is not a new disease but that the potential for this condition has always existed.

CHD was not recognized until the beginning of the last century as a medical phenomenon in its own right. There are two famous descriptions of Angina (the chest pain associated with CHD); that by Edward Hyde (1609–1674) writing about the symptoms suffered by his father, and that by the physician, Dr William Heberden (1710–1801). The chest pain associated with CHD was described and given the name Angina Pectoris by Heberden in a paper published in the Medical Transactions of the College of Physicians in 1772. Heberden appeared not to relate this pain to the heart considering the breast a more likely source of this pectoral pain. He was puzzled too by the intermittent nature of the pain and by the fact that his patients appeared well between episodes. Fortunately for the sufferers he attended, Heberden indicated that bleeding, vomiting and purging were not useful for treating this disorder (Khan and Mehta, 2002). The cardiologist William Osler (1849–1919) took a rather different direction and suggested that angina was a syndrome. It took another cardiologist James B Herrick (1861–1954) to conclude in 1912 not only that a gradual narrowing of the coronary arteries was a possible cause of angina, but this narrowing, even when severe, did not necessarily lead to death.

Bartley (1985) used the Registrar General's annual statistical reviews and the Reports of the Chief Medical Officer to develop a sociological and historical re-reading of CHD. She suggests a conceptual framework showing how, between the two World Wars, CHD came to be seen as a disease associated with affluence and then, post World War II, as a pandemic. This is discussed in more detail below.

Changes during 1921 in the International Classification of Diseases (ICD) and of medical diagnostic practice led to a rapid increase in the numbers of deaths classified as 'degenerative disease of the circulatory system'. By 1927 theories about angina and the relationship of angina to degenerative disease of the coronary arteries had begun to be accepted leading to further changes in ICD coding rules in 1929 so death certificates stating 'myocardial degeneration with arteriosclerosis' were coded specifically as heart disease, allowing the heart to become a primary organ with an associated disease process. From this change Bartley (1985) suggests a conceptual framework had been established for a major cause of death associated with degeneration and failure of the heart due to either, 'sclerotic' and 'fatty' changes, or a blockage in the coronary arteries. This allowed CHD to be attributed to fats (cholesterol) in the blood or deposited in the lining of the coronary arteries; and for theories on diet, physical activity and other aspects of lifestyle to be used to account for CHD development. The impetus for prevention of CHD could then be placed on the individual. CHD began to be viewed as a disease of 'affluence' and 'modern living', as many of the identified risk factors were viewed as 'more typical' of the middle classes.

It became clear in the post World War II period that CHD was also a social phenomenon. During the 1950s, psychiatric opinion suggested that patients with CHD had strongly aggressive tendencies. This opinion influenced the work of Rosenman (1978), who suggested that a uniquely modern 'stress' could play a significantly causal role and that a particular cluster of behavioural traits (named Type A Behaviour Pattern [TABP]) preceded CHD in men and women aged less than 60 years. Individuals with TABP were characterized by enhanced aggressiveness, drive, a chronic sense of urgency and striving, either by preference or necessity, to accomplish more, despite an ever increasing lack of time.

The TABP reinforced a male gender stereotype of CHD that by 1950 had already begun to dominate. The incidence of CHD in women aged less than 60 years was demonstrably lower than that of men and in order to understand and explain these differences investigations into women's personality and stress levels were made. Waldron (1978) proposed that TABP was more prevalent in men than women, which contributed to men's higher rates of premature morbidity and mortality from CHD, and that the sex differences in behaviour patterns appeared to reflect inherited sex differences in aggressiveness and socialization. Women with TABP, Waldron suggested, were more likely to be employed, more likely to seek employment and less likely to leave a job once employed.

Theories of TABP appear to have been absorbed into a common consciousness. The image conjured is of a relatively young and aggressive business man who is always rushing about. Until the late 1980s this image was perceived by both health professionals and lay people as the 'typical' heart attack candidate. Admission protocols in many coronary care units at this time had age policies so that patients over the age of 65 years would not be admitted, effectively ensuring that women – who typically suffer MI around ten years later in life than men – were seldom admitted to such specialist units. Images of coronary care units filled with middle aged men may then have influenced lay health beliefs, as well as approaches to both clinical and social research. However, as the next section explores, a new understanding of the aetiology of CHD began to develop in conjunction with new sociological discourses around the relationship of CHD with socio-economic status, lifestyle, and gender differences.

Professional accounts of coronary heart disease: gendered, social, and moral

In 1991 Healy wrote an editorial in the *New England Journal of Medicine* arguing that 'the problem is to convince both the lay and medical sectors that CHD is also a women's disease, not a man's disease in disguise' (Healy, 1991, p. 275). Women had been systematically excluded from many studies of CHD, a stance justified by the difficulties associated with recruiting younger fertile women or older women with associated co-morbidities to clinical trials. Most studies underpinning the understanding and interventions on CHD have been carried out on exclusively male populations. It has been suggested that by taking white middle aged males as the reference point, and treating gender as just another variable, researchers have them-selves been influenced by the social nature of CHD. This has reinforced the image of CHD as a disease of white men, result-ing in a cycle of comparative neglect – in terms of research and treatment – in women, older people, and other ethnic groups (Khan, 1993). By excluding females as experimental subjects, Rosser (1992) suggests that several areas of biomedicine are biased or flawed. For example, the lack of female participants can lead to faulty experimental designs and the data interpreted using language or ideas constricted by patriarchal values. These flaws and bias, suggests Rosser, are allowed to become part of mainstream science and are perpetuated because most scien-tists are men who do not detect or acknowledge such bias.

Women's experiences of CHD – whilst not homogenous – differ from that of men in terms of presentation, recovery from acute events, morbidity and mortality. Pre-menopausal women experience less morbidity and mortality associated with CHD than do men of a similar age. The accepted biomedical explan-ation points to the protective influence of the ovarian hor-mones in women (Volterrani et al., 1995). However McKinlay (1996) proposed that the lower rates of mortality and mor-bidity from CHD are not indicative necessarily of a reduced prevalence in younger women, but rather, the result of how social statistics are produced. McKinlay argues that to become a statistic two factors need to be in place. First the individual must recognize symptoms and access care; second the gate-keeper for the health system must recognize the condition correctly and apply the correct label. Only when the individ-ual is successful on both counts do the symptoms become a disease and, therefore, a health statistic.

Presentation of CHD symptoms is problematic in that women do not necessarily present with 'typical' symptoms.

Women commonly report experiencing chest pain, however there are a number of reasons for chest pain in women many of which are not cardiac in origin. The language and descriptors women use to describe their chest pain are also more likely to include descriptive accounts of feelings rather than factual descriptions of the location and intensity of pain (Albarran et al., 2000). Women are more likely to describe the pain as pressure, heaviness or tightness and less likely to describe the pain as located in the centre or left of the chest (Milner et al., 1999). Other symptoms also differ by gender with women significantly more likely to report throat pain, neck pain, jaw pain, mid-back pain, nausea and/or vomiting, dyspnoea, palpitations, indigestion and fatigue; symptoms that may be indicative of other long-term conditions such as arthritis or Type II diabetes (Milner et al., 1999; Philpott et al., 2001).

Not only do women present with different symptoms when compared with men but their social circumstances also tend to differ. For example, women tend to be significantly older than men at the time of an acute cardiac event and therefore more likely to be retired (Radley et al., 1998). In comparison to men, women are also less likely to be white (Young and Kahana, 1993), more likely to be unmarried or living alone, possibly as a result of being widowed (Young and Kahana, 1993). Socioeconomically women who present tend to come from poorer backgrounds (Radley et al., 1998) and have attained a lower level of educational achievement (Young and Kahana, 1993).

Recovery from acute cardiac events and invasive procedures such as percutaneous transluminal angioplasty and coronary artery surgery also differs between men and women. After discharge women are more likely to report cardiac related symptoms, functional disability, anxiety and depression (Young and Kahana, 1993). Women are also less likely to attend or complete hospital based cardiac rehabilitation programmes (Radley et al., 1998).

Cardiac rehabilitation programmes, which form the cornerstone of the National Service Framework for Coronary Heart Disease (DH, 2000), however, do not always meet women's needs. Part of the difficulty facing planners of such programmes is the incomplete theoretical understanding of the meaning of an acute cardiac event to the individual. Without such a conceptual framework, nurses and other health professionals working within acute and rehabilitation settings may find their efforts are less effective. Differences in the levels of take up are not just gendered however; older people and people from minority ethnic groups also tend not to take up any cardiac rehabilitation offered. Many studies have focused on the barriers to take up, however it remains true that services do not always meet the individual's perceptions of need and are often delivered at a time and place that is difficult for individuals to access (Lockyer, 2000; Lockyer and Bury, 2002; White, 2000).

Professional accounts of CHD tend to rely heavily on a biomedical discourse, using empirical data that is often, but not always, removed from its social context. Physicians themselves claim that their decisions are purely technical judgements devoid of moral and social content. Hughes and Griffiths (1996) explored these issues through the examination of tape recorded data from angiography conferences, in which cardiologists presented cases to a cardiac surgeon who then had to decide whether to accept the patients for surgery or not. They concluded that although there were discussions as to the technical feasibility of the surgery, the doctors themselves moved between technical and social discourse frames, with a tendency to move beyond technical calculations of risk to consider the 'deserving' characteristics of patients and associated moral agendas. Hughes and Griffiths concluded that because medical practitioners talk in both clinical and everyday moral frameworks there is often ambiguity about which one they are operating in. This overlap between technical discourse dealing with risk and moral discourse dealing with character, the authors suggest, allows the medical practitioners to act to their perceptions of 'deservingness' while accounting for their actions in terms of medical benefit.

Although professional accounts of CHD can be viewed mainly as biomedical discourses, professional actions do not operate within a vacuum and it is clear that while the gendered nature of CHD is acknowledged by health professionals, it is often made to be the patient's problem. Accounts about delay and poor take up of cardiac rehabilitation focus heavily on who does not take up the services and why, but there does not often appear to be within these accounts a recognition of the meaning of CHD to the individuals who are experiencing it and the consequences of this for practice.

Lay accounts of coronary heart disease: acute discourses on chronic diseases

Lay accounts of CHD are inexplicably linked to overarching lay concepts about health. Bury (2005) outlines how sociological research on lay concepts of health and illness identifies complexities and sophistication about medical messages which are translated and reconciled with other knowledge and experience of life; developing into a common consciousness. Blaxter's (1990) classic discussion of lay beliefs indicated that health could be defined negatively as in the absence of disease, functionally as in the ability to cope with everyday activities, or positively as fitness and well-being.

There is also, Bury (2005) indicates, an addition to this picture. Health has a moral dimension, it reflects the adoption and maintenance of a healthy lifestyle, but also how people respond to and deal with their illness. Illness may devalue an identity if the cause is stigmatizing (such as smoking or sexual activity). There are a number of physical and mental conditions that attract a stigma and are associated with negative attributes (see, for example, Chapters 8, 10 and 11). Historically there have been distinctions made between a long-term stigmatizing illness such as tuberculosis or epilepsy and a long-term non stigmatizing illness such as heart disease or diabetes (Peroni, 1981). Conditions once diagnosed may carry a label with them through which individuals may accept an altered identity and lifestyle. When a stigma is attached the stigmatized person may not be held responsible for what is imputed, they may however be denied the ordinary privileges of social life. For a relatively long time CHD was immune from this stigmatizing process, with Sontag (1991) suggesting that compared with HIV/AIDS or some forms of cancer, CHD was not shameful. However, it may be argued that a construction of CHD as morally neutral can no longer be supported (Helman, 1987).

An early study of lay accounts of CHD was undertaken by Davison et al. (1991) who explored lay theories of disease occurrence through a series of interviews with men and women living in South Wales. Almost all interviewed were aware of the behavioural risk factors for CHD, particularly smoking, a fatty diet and a lack of exercise. However, knowledge did not lead to a change in behaviour as the respondents used this knowledge in terms of their existing ideas about CHD; that is; they used both knowledge and ideas to assess their own risk as potential coronary candidates. Davison et al., suggested that the development of ideas is a collective activity in which the mass media, scientific data, and reports of illness and death from family, friends and neighbours are all used as explanatory devices for why individuals develop CHD. Respondents in the study of Davison et al., recognized there were uncertainties surrounding coronary candidacy and that for some, developing or not developing CHD was inexplicable, two categories of individuals are used to illustrate this; the fat old 'Uncle Norman' figure who survives into old age despite drinking, smoking and eating far too much and the slim, fit non-smoker who dies suddenly from a heart attack.

Emslie et al. (2001b), in a 1996 study undertaken in Western Scotland, examined 'lay' notions of CHD coupled with an exploration of whether these varied by social class, age or gender. The men and women who participated in Western Scotland gave very similar descriptions of the coronary candidates to Davison's Welsh participants. However Emslie et al., found some important modifications. The first of these was the realization that, when asked about heart disease the respondents focused on heart attacks, suggesting that lay accounts of coronary candidature are focused on the 'kind of people likely to have a heart attack' rather than the 'kind of people likely to have heart trouble' as Davison et al. (1991) believed. A second modification outlined by Emslie et al. (2001b) was age. Coronary candidates were described as being around late middle or retirement age, however those dying at a young age were seen as 'unlucky victims' whilst for the elderly it was part of old age. Neither the young nor the old were viewed as coronary candidates in the sense that their deaths or heart attacks would be explained through a notion of candidature.

The third modification identified was gender, in that whenever specific candidates were mentioned they were always men; women were invisible in lay accounts of CHD.

Family history (the number, closeness of relationships and age of relatives affected) is also an integral part of many lay accounts of CHD (Hunt et al., 2000; Hunt et al., 2001). However, although physicians and epidemiologists agree that this is relevant, lay interpretations of family history differ from biomedical ones. Hunt et al. (2000), for example, note that lay accounts of 'early death' from CHD differ according to socio-economic status with those in the lowest socio-economic groups being willing to ascribe deaths at a much younger age to 'old age'. People with large numbers of relatives who had CHD did not necessarily feel themselves at risk on account of their family history, as they saw distinct differences between themselves and those relatives who were ill or had died. The study of Davison et al.'s (1991) also demonstrates how individuals' perceptions of risk for CHD acknowledges behavioural factors such as smoking but, when looking for common sense causal explanations for why they themselves developed CHD, they may look else where for a cause. It would appear that behavioural risk factors are too close to home for most people when they are looking for a cause. French et al. (2005) interviewed men and women within a week of their MI and found most actively searching for an explanation of their MI. The most common causal attributions for blame were stress and heredity, not behaviour. Participants' focused on single rather than multiple causes for their MI. French et al., suggest that in studies which ask individuals about their beliefs on causes for their MI the question answered is 'why now?' not 'why?'. They argue that, for many participants, the attributions they highlight after an acute event are the triggers for that event not the factors underlying the chronic process (CHD) that eventually yielded the result (MI).

This interplay between acute and chronic illness models is explored in two studies. Horowitz et al. (2004) interviewed nine women and ten men suffering with congestive heart failure. The results highlight that individuals with heart failure tend to understand their illness in terms of an acute model of chronic illness. The symptoms were viewed as acute manifestations of their heart problems not as something indicative of an underlying chronic illness. This lack of understanding of CHD as a long-term illness in lay accounts means that individuals may perceive CHD, in the form of a MI, as a quick and painless way to die as compared to a lingering and painful death from an illness such as cancer. Emslie et al. (2001a) found few respondents gave narratives of CHD as a long-term condition, the only exceptions being those given by women about female relatives.

The desire shown in a number of lay discourses to avoid self blame for developing CHD indicates that CHD itself now has a degree of censure attached to it. From the early theories about cholesterol and fats, to the identification of behavioural risk factors such as smoking, poor diet and a lack of exercise, individuals may now be labelled as responsible for their health. However, as lay accounts assimilate these biomedical theories, there has developed the desire by individuals to explain and justify their lifestyle and demonstrate their worthiness (Lockyer, 2000).

The studies reviewed suggest that CHD is not perceived by lay people as a long-term condition. However, few studies have used a model of chronic illness to explore CHD. One such study is that by Lockyer (2000) – which explored women's experiences of diagnosis and treatment of CHD – in which Bury's (1991) model of biographical disruption (see also Chapter 1) was used to examine women's experience of CHD (see Figure 5.1). In this study 29 women aged between 51 and 82 years, with an average age of 68 years were interviewed. Twenty-seven of the women were white, one was Chinese and one came from the Philippines.

Initial disruption of illness
↓
Processes of explanation and legitimation
↓
Treatment and adaptation

Figure 5.1   Bury's model of biographical disruption
Source: Adapted from Bury, 1991, pp. 452–453.

A central tenet of Lockyer's research was that women's experiences of CHD could be explored within the context of a long-term condition and, as such, it would be possible to compare similarities in their experience of CHD with the experience described in sociological accounts of other long-term conditions. To this end the interview schedule and analysis followed the model described by Bury (1991). However, throughout the interviews it became clear that although this model held true for some of the women interviewed, for others there were acute and life threatening aspects in the experience of CHD that had little in common with other types of long-term conditions.

Sociological research into other types of long-term conditions has shown that the onset of a chronic illness may be vague and insidious. Most of the women in this study experienced a similar onset that evolved as the disease progressed. A small number of the women claimed they had no symptoms at all until their first MI. The commonest early symptoms in women with CHD are shortness of breath on exercise, tiredness, feelings of tightness or a weight in the chest, and tingling and numbness in the jaw or arm. Many of the women interviewed complained of such vague symptoms at the beginning of their illness but most wrote their symptoms off as normal for 'a woman of their age', as did some of their doctors.

Health is often viewed as an absence of disease or an absence of symptoms and this attitude was clearly demonstrated in the interviews. In this respect CHD was no different from other illnesses. Symptom free women regarded themselves as healthy, despite the fact that they all needed to adjust their lifestyles in order to remain symptom free. Overall it appeared that the majority of women in Lockyer's study attempted to keep control over the events in their lives and care for their own health through a variety of measures including denial of their symptoms, resting, self medication with antacids or over the counter analgesics, or by ascribing any new symptoms to other causes, such as arthritis, which were already diagnosed and under the care of their doctor. Women reacted to their symptoms in terms of their knowledge about their health, life cycle and health beliefs. Their reactions to CHD were influenced by their age, previous life events (e.g., ill health or death of their parents, siblings, children, spouse and friends) and their own concept of their social and domestic role. The fear about CHD expressed by the women was associated with having an acute episode such as an MI and being disabled in the short term or dying; not with the possibility of developing heart failure and having to live with a chronic and debilitating long-term condition.

A significant amount of the sociological literature on CHD has focused around the acute life threatening event or on the experience of heart surgery. It is worth noting here that, historically, invasive tests and treatment for CHD were far more commonly experienced by men than women (Green and Ruffin, 1994), and it may be argued that conclusions made in some of the sociological literature are focused on the meaning of these events for men, not women. However as Frank (1997) notes, the life of a person with a long-term condition is lived substantially outside of the clinical area, with the patient role not encompassing the identity of the ill person, as clinical events are only part of their history. Nonetheless, it was clear from the interviews carried about by Lockyer that the women in this study rated clinical events as very important features in their narratives. Further, that waiting for diagnostic tests, angioplasty, or surgery produced fears about mortality and necessitated a degree of readjustment of perceptions about the quality and quantity of future life.

So, whilst there is a considerable body of sociological literature on lay accounts of health and illness, understanding of how CHD is perceived by lay people remains superficial and the sociological understanding of CHD as a long-term condition remains under explored. The final section of this chapter summarizes the key issues that have been explored and considers the implications of this sociological critique for nurses working with people with CHD.

Nursing people with CHD: the implications of a sociological critique

When researchers ask people about CHD, respondents commonly talk about 'people who are likely to have a heart attack' rather than 'people who are likely to get heart disease'. Research studies also highlight that CHD is not perceived by lay people to be a long-term condition with no cure. This perception is, however, underpinned by health education campaigns which still remain focused on recognizing the symptoms of MI, rather than on the problem of CHD as a long-term condition. The health education campaign aimed at women also remains rather low key despite the National Service Framework for Coronary Heart Disease (DH, 2000) emphasizing the importance of prevention of CHD in women as well as men. This further reinforces the myth of male candidacy for CHD. Lay accounts of inherited or personal risk for CHD also highlight the beginnings of a moral account in which CHD is no longer the badge of honour for a man who work hard until he drops but, rather, the result of a feckless lifestyle where the individual smokes, drinks, eats a poor diet and does not exercise.

A sociological approach suggests that nurses working in primary care, cardiac rehabilitation and acute cardiac care need to recognize that they work within a system that espouses 'gender neutral' treatment and care, where gender neutral usually means 'designed in the first instance to meet the needs of white middle aged men'. To be effective, nurses need to understand the gendered nature of CHD as well as the differences associated with ethnicity and age. Arguably, this needs to be undertaken within a conceptual framework of CHD as a long-term condition particularly since the evidence suggests that lay discourses on CHD do not acknowledge the potential for CHD to lead to extreme levels of disability.

Lay and professional discourses of CHD focus on acute events that are potentially fatal. Whilst nurses and other health professionals understand that CHD is a long-term condition their own discourses often do not have this as a central tenet. The focus is mainly on treating acute dramatic episodes which, if treated promptly, can reduce levels of morbidity and mortality. However, for those concerned with the prevention of CHD and the long-term care needs of those who already have the condition, this is only part of the story. And, of course, for many nurses working outside of acute cardiac or accident and emergency units it is the chronic nature of CHD that is their primary concern.

Until recently the comparative neglect of those with congestive heart failure meant there was also a lack of palliative care for those in the end stages of their lives (also see Chapter 4 for a discussion of palliative care for people with Chronic Obstructive Pulmonary Disease [COPD]). Women, older people and minority ethnic patients were socially pathologized for not taking up cardiac rehabilitation services. These services, while offered with good intentions, were often provided with very little insight as to the relevance of the services for those groups. Services were often not patient-centred and health education the same for all, whether it was relevant or not.

CHD is gendered; the system that diagnoses, refers, treats and rehabilitates individuals was designed for and is based upon the experiences of men. As Healy (1991) has argued, for a woman to receive treatment she needs to present as a man or her symptoms will not be recognized. Although it is now acknowledged that large numbers of women experience CHD, it is fair to suggest that decisions about diagnosis, treatment and management will be made against the background of the prototypical male patient. Equally such decisions are often made in the light of health professionals' experiences of therapeutic regimes designed for and monitored in terms of the needs of male patients (Lockyer and Bury, 2002).

CHD will remain as a major source of mortality and morbidity in the United Kingdom and other similarly developed countries and as acute episodes are treated more successfully there will be larger numbers of older people living with CHD as a long-term condition. How their CHD progresses and how they experience their disease will, in part, depend on how nurses and other health professionals take up the challenge.

References

Albarran, J.M., B. Durham, G. Chappel, J. Dwight and J. Gowers, 'Are manual gestures, verbal descriptors and pain radiation as reported by patients reliable indicators of myocardial infarction? Preliminary findings and implications', *Intensive and Critical Care Nursing*, 16 (2000) 98–110.

Allender S., V. Peto, P. Scarborough, A. Boxer and M. Rayner, *Coronary Heart Disease Statistics 2006 Edition* (London: British

Heart Foundation Statistics Database, 2006) http:www.heartstats. org (last accessed 28 December 2006).

Bartley M., 'Coronary heart disease and the public health 1850–1983', *Sociology of Health and Illness*, 7: 3 (1985) 289–313.

Bury M., *Health and Illness* (Cambridge Malden: Polity, 2005).

Bury M., 'The sociology of chronic illness: a review of research and prospects', *Sociology of Health and Illness*, 13 (1991) 451–468.

Blaxter M., *Health and Lifestyles* (London/New York: Routledge, 1990).

Davison C., G. Davey Smith and S. Frankel, 'Lay epidemiology and the prevention paradox: the implications of coronary candidacy for health education', *Sociology of Health and Illness*, 13: 1 (1991) 1–19.

Department of Health (DH), *National Service Framework for Coronary Heart Disease Modern Standards and Service Models* (London: Department of Health, London, 2000).

Emslie C., K. Hunt and G. Watt, ' "I'd rather go with a heart attack than drag on": lay images of heart disease and the problems they present for primary and secondary prevention', *Coronary Health Care*, 5 (2001a) 25–32.

Emslie C., K. Hunt and G. Watt, 'Invisible women? The importance of gender in lay beliefs about heart problems', *Sociology of Health and Illness*, 23: 2 (2001b) 203–233.

Frank A.W., 'Illness as moral occasion: restoring agency to ill people', *Health*, 1: 2 (1997) 131–148.

French D.P., E. Maissi and T.M. Marteau, 'The purpose of attributing cause: beliefs about the causes of myocardial infarction', *Social Science and Medicine*, 60 (2005) 1411–1421.

Green L.A., and M.T. Ruffin, 'A closer examination of sex bias in the treatment of Ischemic cardiac disease', *The Journal of Family Practice*, 39: 4 (1994) 331–336.

Healy B., 'The Yentl syndrome', *New England Journal of Medicine*, 325 (1991) 274–276.

Helman C.G., 'Heart disease and the cultural construction of time: the type A behaviour pattern as a western culture-bound syndrome', *Social Science and Medicine*, 25 (1987) 969–979.

Horowitz C.R., S.B. Rein and H. Leventhal, 'A story of maladies, misconceptions and mishaps: effective management of heart failure', *Social Science and Medicine*, 58: 3 (2004) 631–643.

Hughes D., and L. Griffiths, ' "But if you look at the coronary anatomy...": risk and rationing in cardiac surgery', *Sociology of Health and Illness*, 18: 2 (1996) 172–197.

Hunt K., C. Davison, C. Emslie and G. Ford, 'Are perceptions of a family history of heart disease related to health-related attitudes and behaviour?', *Health Education Research*, 15: 2 (2000) 131–143.

Hunt K., C. Emslie and G. Watt, 'Lay constructions of a family history of heart disease: potential for misunderstandings in the clinical encounter?', *The Lancet*, 357 (2001) 1168–1171.

Khan I.A., and N.J. Mehta, 'Initial historical descriptions of the angina pectoris', *The Journal of Emergency Medicine*, 22: 3 (2002) 295–298.

Khan K.T., 'Where are the women in the studies of coronary heart disease?', *British Medical Journal*, 306 (1993) 1145–1146.

Lockyer L., *The Experience of Women in the Diagnosis and Treatment of Coronary Heart Disease*, PhD Thesis (London: University of London, 2000).

Lockyer L., and M. Bury, 'The construction of a modern epidemic: the implications for women of the gendering of coronary heart disease', *Journal of Advanced Nursing*, 39: 5 (2002) 432–440.

McKinlay J.B., 'Some contributions from the social system to gender inequalities in heart disease', *Journal of Health and Social Behavior*, 37 (1996) 1–26.

Mackay J., and G. Mensah (2004) *The Atlas of Heart Disease and Stroke* (Geneva: WHO, 2004) http://www.who.int/cardiovascular_diseases/resources/atlas/en/ (last accessed 11 December 2007).

Milner K.A., M. Funk, S. Richards, R.M. Wilmes, V. Vaccarino and H.M. Krumholz, 'Gender differences in symptom presentation associated with coronary heart disease', *The American Journal of Cardiology*, 84 (1999) 396–399.

Peroni F., 'The status of chronic illness', *Social Policy and Administration*, 15: 1 (1981) 43–53.

Philpott S., P.M. Boynton, G. Feder and H. Hemingway, 'Gender differences in descriptions of angina symptoms and health problems immediately prior to angiography: the ACRE study', *Social Science and Medicine*, 52 (2001) 1565–1575.

Radley A., A. Grove, S. Wright and H. Thurston, 'Problems of women compared with those of men following myocardial infarction', *Coronary Health Care*, 2 (1998) 202–209.

Rosenman R., 'Introduction', in T.M. Dembroski, S.M. Weiss, J.L. Shields, S.G. Haynes and M. Feinleib (eds), *Coronary Prone Behavior* (New York Heidelberg Berlin: Springer – Verlag, 1978).

Rosser S.V., 'Gender bias in clinical research: the difference it makes', in A.J. Dan (ed.), *Reframing Women's Health. Multidisciplinary*

Research and Practice (London: Thousand Oaks; New Delhi: Sage Publications, 1992).

Sharp I., *Coronary Heart Disease: Are Women Special?* (London: National Forum for Coronary Heart Disease Prevention, 1994).

Sontag S., *Illness as Metaphor. AIDS and Its Metaphors* (London: Penguin Books, 1991).

Volterrani M., G. Rosano, A. Coats, C. Beale and P. Collins, 'Estrogen acutely increases peripheral blood flow in postmenopausal women', The *American Journal of Medicine*, 99 (1995) 119–122.

Waldron I., 'Sex differences in the coronary-prone behavior pattern', in T.M. Dembroski, S.M. Weiss, J.L. Shields, S.G. Haynes and M. Feinleib (eds), *Coronary Prone Behavior* (New York Heidelberg Berlin: Springer – Verlag, 1978).

White A.K., *Men Making Sense of Their Chest Pain, PhD Thesis* (Manchester: University of Manchester, 2000).

Young R.F., and E. Kahana, 'Gender, recovery from late life heart attack, and medical care', *Women and Health*, 20: 1 (1993) 11–31.

6 Policy and practice for diabetes care

Cathy E. Lloyd and
T. Chas Skinner

Introduction

Diabetes, one of the most common long-term conditions, is a major health concern of the twenty-first century, with the incidence and prevalence of this condition increasing rapidly (DH, 2001). This has huge consequences for all sections of the health service, as the care of diabetes and its complications, which include eye disease, heart disease, and renal failure, is carried out within both primary and secondary care.

Ideally, the care of diabetes requires a dual approach with people with the condition caring for themselves on a day-to-day basis, in partnership with a number of different health care professionals. However, this is not without its difficulties and the link between sub-optimal self-care and poor outcomes in diabetes is now widely accepted. The wide range of self-care behaviours (including blood glucose monitoring, medication taking, dietary monitoring and physical activity) expected to be performed by the individual with diabetes is often considered to be intrusive, time-consuming and burdensome. Research has demonstrated that there is a wide variability in the degree to which those individuals carry out these self-care activities. This chapter considers current policy and practice in diabetes care, including the implementation of the National Service Framework (NSF) for diabetes, and the implications of this for those working with people with diabetes. The focus here is on adults with the condition; separate policy and practice guidelines have been developed for children and young people (e.g., see *Making Every Young Person with Diabetes Matter*, DH, 2007). However, children with diabetes have significant difficulties in maintaining optimal levels of blood sugar and this has important implications for practice. Children spend about a quarter of their time in school, however guidelines for the management of diabetes in schools, and adequate support for both children and their teachers remains poor. Children and their families may find the often unpredictable nature of diabetes (e.g., during growth periods or adolescence) difficult, with fear of low blood sugars (hypoglycaemia) being a major concern. Diabetes UK have recently launched a new advocacy service to help people understand what health care they should expect to receive and one of the topics covered concerns the care of diabetes in schools. However, further research is clearly warranted in order to better understand the needs and experiences of children and young people with diabetes and how those needs can be supported through clinical practice. This chapter examines how nurses and other health care professionals in both primary and secondary care settings work with people with diabetes in order to optimize care. In particular, an empowerment approach to care will be considered and the implications of this for nursing practice discussed.

Strategies for care

Across the world the incidence and prevalence of diabetes is increasing (DH, 2001). At the same time the impact on all concerned – including the individual with diabetes and the health care professionals involved in their care – rises exponentially. Diabetes brings with it an increased risk of a range of potentially devastating complications including blindness, renal failure, cardiovascular disease and diabetic neuropathy. Psychological problems, such as depression and anxiety, are also much more common in people with diabetes compared to those without (Lloyd, 2000; Lustmann et al., 1996, 1998). Having a chronic condition such as diabetes also has implications for employment opportunities, social and personal relationships, as well as the possibility of disability and the often accompanying stigma and social exclusion.

The NSF for diabetes, published in 2001, set out minimum standards of care for those with this condition (DH, 2001), and this was followed by a delivery strategy for the NSF (DH, 2003). The NSF for diabetes had important implications for both people with diabetes and the health care professionals involved in their care. A partnership approach to care was advocated, but this implied knowledge and understanding of diabetes and how to achieve optimum standards of care on both sides. A wide range of health care personnel could potentially be involved in this care, including physicians, nurses, health care assistants, dieticians, and podiatrists, working alongside the individual with the condition itself as well as their family. New roles within diabetes care have also been advocated, with the development of the Diabetes Care Technician and the expert patient programme (Banks, 2005). The NSF delivery strategy proposed undertaking a local workforce skills profile of staff involved in the care of people with diabetes, as well as developing education and training programs (DH, 2001). The UK government body, Skills for Health, have also developed competency frameworks in order to influence the training of health care professionals involved in diabetes care (www.skillsforhealth.org.uk) (last accessed 15 September 2008). Forty-five competencies have been identified for diabetes care, linked to the Key Skills Framework to which every National Health Service (NHS) job must be mapped. These new standards have serious implications for the education and training of health service workers.

An empowerment approach to diabetes care

A partnership approach to care, as advocated in the NSF for diabetes, implies that health care professionals and the person with diabetes should work together towards commonly agreed goals. A joint approach to diabetes care was proposed in the NSF, which entailed the person with diabetes working with the health care professionals in order to optimize care. The third of the twelve standards set out in the NSF is of particular importance here (see Box 6.1).

> **Box 6.1**   Standard 3: empowering people with diabetes
>
> All children, young people and adults with diabetes will receive a service which encourages partnership in decision-making, supports them in managing their diabetes and helps them adopt and maintain a healthy lifestyle. This will be reflected in an agreed and shared care plan in an appropriate format and language. When appropriate, parents and carers should be fully engaged in this process.
>
> *Source*: DH, 2001, p. 5.

The principle of empowerment in diabetes care is based upon people taking more control of their care, both for themselves as individuals, and also for others being involved in determining local services and priorities (Anderson and Funnell, 2000). Recent guidelines for children and young people advocate the promotion 'of self-care and empowerment via measures such as education.' (DH, 2007, p. 49). An empowerment approach to care takes into account social, psychological and environmental factors are well as medical ones. Hiscock (2001) has identified a set of factors that contribute to a positive experience in diabetes care which include:

- A friendly, warm and 'equal' approach to the person with diabetes
- A willingness to understand the impact of diabetes on other aspects of the individual's life and lifestyle
- A 'partnership approach' to treating the condition
- A willingness to make time to discuss issues and answer questions
- A proactive approach to making referrals to other health care professionals. (Adapted from Hiscock et al., 2001)

Anderson and Funnell (2000) have compared two models of diabetes care, which are reproduced in the Table 6.1. They compare an empowerment model with what they call a 'traditional model' of care, and identify the differences in styles of care in terms of providing diabetes education. Diabetes education, usually provided by nurses, is the cornerstone of diabetes care and includes not only knowledge and information dissemination but skills and confidence building in order for each individual to feel able to carry out diabetes self-care activities.

Table 6.1 Two models of diabetes education

The empowerment model	The traditional model
1. Diabetes is a bio-psychosocial illness.	1. Diabetes is a physical Illness.
2. Relationship of provider and patient is democratic and based on shared expertise.	2. Relationship of provider and patient is authoritarian based on provider expertise.
3. Problems and learning needs are usually identified by the patient.	3. Problems and learning needs are usually identified by professional.
4. Patient is viewed as problem solver and caregiver, that is, professional acts as a resource and helps the patient set goals and develop a self-management plan.	4. Professional is viewed as problem solver and caregiver, that is, professional responsible for diagnosis, and outcome.
5. Goal is to enable patients to make informed choices. Behavioural strategies are used to help patients experiment with behaviour changes of their choosing. Behaviour changes that are not adopted are viewed as learning tools to provide new information that can be used to develop future plans and goals.	5. Goal is behaviour change. Behavioural strategies are used to increase compliance with recommended treatment. A lack of compliance is viewed as a failure of patient and provider.
6. Behaviour changes are internally motivated.	6. Behaviour changes are externally motivated.
7. Patient and professional are powerful.	7. Patient is powerless, professional is powerful.

Source: Anderson and Funnel, 2000, p. 43.

© 2005, American Diabetes Association. From the Art of Empowerment 2nd edn. Reprinted with permission from *The American Diabetes Association*.

Whilst using an empowerment approach to diabetes care may seem fairly straightforward to some practitioners, given the huge variability in patient need, type of diabetes care regimen and external factors that might influence self-care, the implications can be daunting. It implies that during each consultation between the person with diabetes and a health care professional a dialogue should take place during which these factors can be taken into account. Given the time constraints as well as the range of communication skills required, this might be challenging to say the least.

Diabetes education

In order to become equally involved in diabetes care it can be argued that greater knowledge and understanding of diabetes is essential. The National Institute for Health and Clinical Excellence (NICE) has recommended that all people with diabetes should be offered structured education (NICE, 2003). The education should be provided by an 'appropriately trained multidisciplinary team to groups of people with diabetes, unless group work is considered unsuitable for an individual' (NICE, 2003, p. 4). NICE advocates that patient education should be tailored to meet specific needs and must be 'accessible to the broadest range of people, taking into account culture, ethnicity, disability and geographical issues' (NICE, 2003, p. 4). Given the variability of diabetes knowledge and understanding in health care services in general, the promotion of structured education for people with diabetes by NICE has been broadly welcomed (NICE, 2003). The most recent guidance on this however, did not consider education for the families and carers of people with diabetes, a vital component of diabetes care. The exception to this is the guidance for children and young people, where the need to involve the family in diabetes care has been acknowledged (DH, 2007).

Not only is knowledge of diabetes vital, the confidence or perceived self-efficacy to be able to carry out all the various aspects of self-management is equally important. Self-efficacy theory (Bandura, 1977) is attracting increasing interest in relation to understanding individual health behaviour. Self-efficacy measurement instruments can provide an indication of an individual's perception of their ability to perform particular activities. In diabetes, performing specific activities (e.g., blood glucose monitoring), dietary modification and medication adherence is crucial. The value of self-efficacy theory to guide health professional interventions, or, of self-efficacy instruments to demonstrate the success of educational interventions, is becoming more widely researched (Barlow and Sturt, 2002; Lorig et al., 1999). Currently, a number of initiatives in the United Kingdom are promoting an empowerment approach to diabetes management, placing the emphasis of care on the person with diabetes in conjunction with Diabetes Specialist Nurse education. One of the most well-known initiatives, Diabetes Education and Self-Management for Ongoing and Newly Diagnosed (DESMOND) is supported by Diabetes UK and works from the principles of empowerment and a partnership approach to diabetes care (DESMOND, 2004). The DESMOND collaborative has identified a number of responsibilities of health care professionals working with individuals with Type 2 diabetes (see Box 6.2).

Box 6.2 The DESMOND collaborative: responsibilities for health care professionals

- Ensuring individuals with diabetes and their carers are provided with honest, up to date, evidence-based information regarding the causes, effects and options for the management of Type 2 diabetes
- Ensuring that those living with Type 2 diabetes are aware of their specific individual ongoing health risks for developing the complications of diabetes
- Providing systems of care which are accessible to everyone
- Ensuring, that everyone, regardless of how they decide to manage their diabetes, is treated with the utmost respect and unconditional positive regard
- Ensuring that individuals with diabetes are supported in the development of the general self-management skills (e.g., goal setting, action planning and problem solving) necessary for the effective management of a chronic condition
- Ensuring that individuals with diabetes are supported in the development of the general diabetes specific self-management necessary for the effective management of Type 2 diabetes
- Ensuring that individuals are supported in managing their emotional responses to the diagnosis of diabetes, its impact on their life and the impact of diabetes complications

Source: Adapted from DESMOND collaborative 2004, pp. 5–7.

DESMOND may not be suitable for all those with diabetes and other programmes of structured education, for example the Diabetes X-Pert Programme (X-Pert Programme, 2008), may be more appropriate in order to meet the needs of individuals with language or cultural barriers. The use of self-efficacy theory in underpinning initiatives such as DESMOND could be argued to divert attention away from structural or social barriers to care. These include poverty, socio-cultural issues, and unequal access to services. Poor communication, lack of understanding or misconceptions about how individuals view their diabetes and the care required are also important factors to take into account when planning and delivering the most appropriate form of diabetes education and care.

A partnership approach?

A partnership approach to diabetes care, with the person with diabetes working together with a range of health care professionals within a multidisciplinary team is recommended by government bodies, Diabetes UK, and many others working within the field of diabetes. However, this may appear to be difficult to attain in some circumstances. In particular, these aims and goals may be difficult to achieve when working with particular sections of the diabetes population. Given the increasing prevalence of diabetes in people from minority ethnic backgrounds, working with and understanding the issues and particular concerns of individuals from minority ethnic backgrounds has become of greater concern.

The risk of diabetes, particularly Type 2 diabetes, is known to be greater in minority ethnic groups, such as in the South Asian communities in the United Kingdom. It is over four times more common and age of onset is earlier (Chowdhury and Lasker, 2002; DH, 2003). There are also a number of particular problems with regard to the management of the condition in this group. In particular cultural and communication difficulties often make appropriate support of self-management of diabetes more difficult (Baradaran and Knill-Jones, 2004; Greenhalgh et al., 1998; Lloyd et al., 2006; Vyas, 2003). For instance, in a recent study by Lloyd et al. (2006) it became clear that written translations of patient information sheets did little to overcome barriers to communication between health care professionals and individuals with diabetes as the majority of those enrolled in the study were unable to read or write any language and used only local dialects that did not have an agreed written form. Many current initiatives in diabetes are mainly focused on people in the United Kingdom who are fluent in English, and little is yet understood about the particular needs of minority ethnic groups (Lloyd et al., 2006). However, a small study recently demonstrated that the use of Asian Support Workers, or Asian Link Workers, markedly improves patient outcomes, in terms of increased knowledge and understanding of their diabetes, improved attendance rates at clinics and at education sessions (Curtis et al., 2003). An understanding of cultural differences is important; however it is vital that difference is not assumed on the basis of appearance or language. Diversity is present within as well as between different cultural groups and an understanding of individual needs and concerns remains key if self-care is to be optimized.

Psychological well-being

Diabetes care is also affected by psychological and emotional well-being and in recent years there has been a heightened interest in psychological well-being and diabetes. Although depressed mood is a common occurrence in both people with and without diabetes, research has shown that it is more common in people with diabetes (Lustman et al., 1996). In the general population, 5–8 per cent of people will be experiencing a major depressive episode at any point in time but it is two to three times more common in people with diabetes compared to those without diabetes (Anderson et al., 2001). In one study in the United Kingdom, 38 per cent of diabetes outpatients reported moderate to severe levels of anxiety or depression (Lloyd et al., 2000). The reason why people with diabetes report higher rates may be linked to the demands of managing a long term condition and the constant demands for self-care required of the individual with diabetes, along with the frequent lack of resources needed to manage diabetes, other aspects of material deprivation and low levels of education.

Psychological well-being impacts on self-care; for example, depressed mood often leads to poor dietary management, lack of physical activity, and poor health behaviours such as increased smoking and alcohol intake. Depressed mood is also associated with an increase in the hormone cortisol which leads to increases in blood glucose levels and thereby poorer glycaemic control. This in turn can lead to an increased risk of developing diabetes complications. Although depression is often undiagnosed and therefore untreated, antidepressant therapy has been shown to be effective and has been found to be associated with improved levels of glycaemic control (Lustman et al., 1998). The NSF for diabetes recognizes that: 'diabetes can have a major impact on the physical, psychological and material well-being of individuals and their families ... [and that it was important to develop] strategies to deal with the psychological consequences of illness' (DH, 2001, p. 22).

NICE have provided a framework in which to organize the provision of services supporting patients/carers and healthcare professionals in identifying and accessing the most effective interventions. A 'stepped-care' model for depression was recommended, as it was recognized that depressed people have different needs, depending on the characteristics of their depression and their personal and social circumstances (see Figure 6.1). According to this model, different responses are required from the health care services depending on the needs of the individual.

However, as reported by Diabetes UK in their State of the Nation report (2005), many people felt the provision of emotional support was still a significant gap in diabetes services, particularly for children, young people and parents (Diabetes UK, 2005). A report published by the DH Diabetes Policy Team (2007) seeks to address specific issues of both physical and psychological wellbeing in children and young people although it remains to be seen whether recommendations are put into practice. Only 39 per cent of people with diabetes reported they had been offered and accessed emotional help and support in recent years (Diabetes UK, 2005).

More recently, the Quality Outcomes Framework (QoF) system now includes diabetes associated depression indicators and guidance (National Diabetes Support Team, 2006). Up to eight

Step 5:	Inpatient care, crisis teams	Risk to life, severe self-neglect	Medication, combined treatments, ECT
Step 4:	Mental health specialists, including crisis teams	Treatment-resistant, recurrent, atypical and psychotic depression, and those at significant risk	Medication, complex psychological interventions, combined treatments
Step 3:	Primary care team, primary care mental health worker	Moderate or severe depression	Medication, psychological interventions, social support
Step 2:	Primary care team, primary care mental health worker	Mild depression	Watchful waiting, guided self-help, computerised CBT, exercise, brief psychological interventions
Step 1:	Gp, practice nurse	Recognition	Assessment

Figure 6.1 The stepped-care model for depression (NICE 2007)

Source: National Institute for Health and Clinical Excellence (NICE) (2007) CG023 Depression (amended): management of depression in primary and secondary care. London: NICE. Available from www.nice.org.uk/GG023. Reproduced with permission.

points on the QoF system are available for general practices that can show they have screened patients with diabetes for depression during the last 15 months using two standard questions:

1. During the last month, have you been bothered by feeling down, depressed or hopeless?
2. During the last month, have you often been bothered by having little interest or pleasure in doing things?

Up to 25 points are available for practices that can show they have made an assessment of severity of depression (in those with a new diagnosis of depression) at the outset of treatment using an assessment tool validated for use in primary care. Although it might be considered problematic to administer screening questionnaires to detect symptoms of depression or other psychological problems in a clinic setting, previous research has indicated that this can be achieved and is often perceived as entirely acceptable by both patients and clinical staff (Lloyd et al., 2000). In this latter study, in which a high response rate was achieved (96 per cent), one third of those who completed a screening questionnaire reported they would be interested in receiving counseling or psychotherapy if it was currently available at the clinic. Those in this group were significantly more likely to have moderate-severe anxiety/depression scores.

Given the plethora of research demonstrating the importance of psychological well-being in those with diabetes, and the official guidance in terms of screening as well as treating psychological problems, this has serious implications for the health care professionals working with those with diabetes. The Diabetes UK State of the Nations report (2005) stated that 'All people with diabetes need access to psychological and emotional support…so that they can manage their condition effectively and reduce the risk of complications' (Diabetes UK, 2005, p. 31). Furthermore, the access to psychological and emotional support should come 'from healthcare professionals with the appropriate skills' (Diabetes UK, 2005, p. 31). In order to meet those needs, however, greater resources need to be invested to increase access to specialist psychological and emotional support for people with diabetes.

Assessing the need for care for psychological problems in primary care is problematic. Health care professionals require training in order to carry out screening, diagnosis and treatment. Alternatively, if screening was considered routine, the multidisciplinary team working with the person with diabetes would either include a health care professional trained in screening techniques or the team would contain a psychologist/psychiatrist who would be able to care for the person with psychological problems.

The person with diabetes

So far this chapter has considered policy and practice for diabetes care from the perspective of health care professionals, but what of the perspectives and experiences of the person with diabetes? Education initiatives such as DESMOND assume a partnership approach to care with the person with diabetes at the centre. They assume that the person with diabetes is willing and/or able to strive for the goal of good glycaemic control through appropriate self-management, the skills for which are imparted through diabetes education and support. These assumptions are built into the NSF for diabetes and other policy/practice recommendations.

Possibly one of the main reasons that the NSF for diabetes sought to push the agenda of empowerment onto health care professionals was a realization that current approaches to diabetes care, in the United Kingdom and around the world are not realizing the outcomes that would be expected based on the development of new drugs and treatment regimens. Most large scale surveys across the world have found that the majority of people with diabetes do not reach or sustain their goals, even with intensive support and when this is available good metabolic control often remains elusive. For some commentators the answer to this problem lies within notions of 'non-adherence' or 'non-compliance'. The concept of compliance implies that the patient is a passive recipient of doctors' orders; the doctor being the person with the knowledge of 'what's best' for the patient. Non-compliance therefore is seen to occur when the patient does not follow doctors' orders and, in the case of diabetes, does not perform recommended self-management behaviour such as testing blood sugars, medication taking and dietary self-management. However, the concept of non-compliance may not necessarily be a helpful one when trying to understand how individuals look after themselves. As Lerner argues, in a review of the literature on non-compliance, using 'labels such as "non-compliant" are invariably judgmental' (Lerner, 1997, p. 1423).

In recent years there has been a further rejection of the notion of non-compliance in favour of 'concordance' (Ferner, 2003). Proponents of concordance argue that this is a far preferable term as it promotes constructive dialogue between patient and health care professional. This dialogue includes discussion of the risks and benefits of any medication taking or other self-care activities, and forms the basis on which any decisions on the part of patient can be made.

For the person with diabetes, concordance with recommendations for self-care may be varied; even though insulin may be injected at the appropriate times, or other diabetes medication taken, this does not mean that other vital aspects of diabetes self-care are performed. One of the most widely used survey instruments to assess the behaviour of people with diabetes is the Summary of Diabetes Self-Care Activities questionnaire (Toobert et al., 2000). Using data from seven studies totalling over 1,800 individuals with diabetes, on average Toobert et al., report the following findings with regards to people with diabetes following their health care professionals' recommendations (see Box 6.3).

Box 6.3   How often do people with diabetes follow their self-care regimen?

People with diabetes report following the different aspects of their self-care regimen for varying degrees of time. They follow their:

- general dietary recommendations about 59 per cent of the time
- specific dietary recommendations about 68 per cent of the time
- exercise recommendations about 34 per cent of the time
- blood glucose testing recommendations about 69 per cent of the time
- medication taking recommendations about 95 per cent of the time
- foot care recommendations about 47 per cent of the time.

Source: Adapted from Toobert et al., 2000.

As Toobert et al., note, this is not 95 per cent of people following their medication taking instructions, but that each person on the whole reports following their recommendations about 95 per cent of the time, or to put it another way, they miss their medication one day in every 20. Other research in medication taking also suggests that people with diabetes (and indeed other long-term conditions) do not take all their medications as recommended by their doctor (Benner et al., 2002; Chapman et al., 2005).

Given the scale of this issue it is unsurprising that there is an abundance of literature on the problems of what has been known as 'compliance' and 'adherence'. At the time of writing, entering the term 'compliance' into PUBMED located 72,784 citations of the word compliance in abstracts and titles, of which 9,524 were reviews and 240 meta-analyses. Using the term 'adherence' resulted in 41,115 citations, of which 4,348 were reviews and 119 were meta-analyses. One recent meta-analysis highlighted the impact of the problem of adherence to medical treatments in a range of randomized trials (Simpson et al., 2006). They concluded that for those with good adherence the risk of death was about half that of individuals with poor adherence. There have also been systematic reviews of the literature with regard to ways of improving adherence to medical treatments.

The Cochrane Library contains three systematic reviews on this matter; one specifically on interventions to improve adherence to medication for type 2 diabetes (Vermeire et al., 2005), and two (one an update of the other) looking at interventions to improve adherence to medication generally (Haynes et al., 2007). However, the conclusions to these reviews provide rather grim reading. Based on a rather limited range of 21 studies Vermeire and colleagues concluded that:

> Current efforts to improve or facilitate adherence of people with type 2 diabetes to treatment recommendations do not show significant effects nor harms. The question whether any intervention enhances adherence to treatment recommendations in type 2 diabetes effectively, thus still remains unanswered. (Vermeire et al., 2007, p. 13)

Even though Haynes and colleagues identified more studies, few were methodological sound, and they concluded that:

> For long term treatments, 26 of 58 interventions reported in 49 RCTs were associated with improvements in adherence, but only 18 interventions led to improvement in at least one treatment outcome. Almost all of the interventions that were effective for long-term care were complex, including combinations of more convenient care, information, reminders, self-monitoring, reinforcement, counseling, family therapy, psychological therapy, crisis intervention, manual telephone follow-up, and supportive care. The diversity, complexity, and uncertain effects of the interventions make generalizations problematic about which interventions work and which don't. Even the most effective interventions did not lead to large improvements in adherence and treatment outcomes. (Haynes et al., 2007, p. 13)

Given the abundance of the literature identified earlier, these results can be only be considered as disappointing at the very best, and further research is clearly needed. As argued previously, the perspective of the person with the long term condition needs to be understood and this should be a key focus of future research. Challenging notions of compliance or adherence to medications, working from the patient's perspective and incorporating issues around empowerment into diabetes care can lead to a re-thinking of ideas about self-care and a greater understanding of why some people take their medications and other people do not.

Challenges to the biomedical model

One of the premises behind the idea of empowerment is to challenge the traditional biomedical view of how diabetes is managed. The notion of adherence is possibly the best example of this, with the World Health Organization defining it as 'the extent to which a person's behaviour – taking medication, following a diet, and/or executing lifestyle changes, corresponds with agreed recommendations from a health care provider' (Sabate, 2003). This definition, as well as the definitions for similar terms used in the literature, such as compliance and concordance, are based upon a clear set of assumptions:

1. There are a clear set of instructions to comply or adhere to
2. That health care professionals agree on what a person should be trying to do
3. That there is agreement about what decisions have been made
4. That health care professionals accurately recall what they tell people with diabetes

A further assumption is that people with diabetes are willing/able to perform all the different self-care behaviours, and that structural or environmental factors do not impact on self-management. In addition, although there are commonly agreed goals or aims of treatment and self-management of diabetes, the pathway to these outcomes is not universally agreed. People with type 2 diabetes are asked to perform a whole range of tasks:

- Reduce fat intake
- Reduce saturated fat intake
- Reduce calorie intake
- Increase fibre intake

- Increase fruit and vegetable intake
- Reduce glycaemic index of food taken
- Take each medication, at the prescribed time, in the right dose
- Quit Smoking
- Increase physical activity
- Monitor urine/blood sugars
- Reduce stress levels
- Increase medication when ill.

Additional self-care behaviours are required for those treating their diabetes with insulin. For example, when blood sugars might be low, blood glucose levels must be checked, and if necessary food should be eaten followed by further checks. This complexity belies the idea that there is a simple set of instructions that individuals with diabetes follow. Research has shown that communicating these instructions for self-management of diabetes is difficult, as with any long term condition, misunderstandings and poor recall after doctor-patient communication are common (Ferner, 2003). Consider the stories from various pharmacists in Box 6.4:

Box 6.4 Stories from pharmacists

An elderly patient who was taking several medications complained to her pharmacist that she was having trouble taking her potassium. The pharmacist asked, 'What seems to be the problem? Are you taking it as instructed?' The patient replied, 'Yes, that's no problem. I take it just like it says on the label: "Take one tablet each morning in water". But I prefer to take my bath at night, not in the morning.'

A nine month-old baby had to be admitted to the hospital with a severe infection because his mother misunderstood the labelled instructions for an antibiotic: 'Take one-half teaspoonful three times a day for infection until all gone.' The mother continued the drug for about three days, until the baby appeared to be getting better. The mother then stopped giving the antibiotic; a super-infection developed and the baby was hospitalised.

A patient returned to the pharmacy complaining of side effects apparently caused by his medication. The patient's records indicated he had been dispensed 30 nitroglycerin patches. Both the pharmacist and physician told him to 'apply one daily'. The patient opened his shirt to reveal 27 nitro patches.

Source: Tindall, Beardsley and Kimberlin, 2001.

Doctor-patient communication

The stories in Box 6.4 reveal high levels of miscommunication between health care professional and patient. There have been many sociological studies of patient – doctor communication (see for example Clark, 1992; Fisher, 1984; May et al., 2004), although few have considered the level of agreement with regards the decisions made between doctors and patients for diabetes care. In a recent study however a comparison of the recollections of diabetes specialist nurses and dietitians with those of the patient was carried out (Parkin and Skinner, 2003). Immediately after an outpatient consultation, both the person with diabetes and the health care professional was asked about what had been decided in the consultation. The responses were then compared and coded into three categories:

1. Complete Agreement – where the topics and specific content were the same;
2. Some Agreement – where either the topics were the same but the specifics differed, or there was any overlap between the topics given by participant and professional;
3. Complete Disagreement – where there was no overlap on the topics given by the participants and professionals.

Patients and professionals completely disagreed with each other on the decisions made in the consultation in 20 per cent of the consultations (Parkin and Skinner, 2003). Although this problem can be improved somewhat by training professionals in communication skills (Parkin et al., 2006; Woodcock and Kinmonth, 2001) the problem remains intransient.

Disagreement with regards the content of the consultations is often thought to be related to poor recall on the part of the patient, although this has rarely been tested out (Page et al., 1981). As a follow up to the previous work cited above (Parkin and Skinner, 2003) consultations between diabetes specialist nurses and dietitians and their patients were audio-recorded, and the decisions being made between the participants were identified. For a decision to be recorded, two criteria had to be met; (i) the health professional, or patient, had to make a clear statement; questions such as 'what do you think about increasing your insulin?' were not considered as advice or a treatment decision; (ii) the statement needed to include an action that either the patient or professional was to undertake. Patient and professional recall of the consultation with regards the actual decisions made were then compared. Both the health care professional and the patient correctly recalled fewer decisions that were made than were identified by the researchers from the audio-tape. Importantly, other decisions 'recalled' by the health care professionals when interviewed, were not identified by the researchers when reviewing the audio-tape; in short the professionals were recalling decisions that had not actually been made (i.e., verbally agreed between health care professional and patient) (Skinner et al., 2007). When providing feedback to the professionals and giving them the chance to review their audio tapes two issues seemed dominant. These were where professionals asked patients questions, but recorded this as a decision, and professionals thinking and even noting something that needs to be done, but not actually verbalizing this.

Not only might there be lack of agreement on treatment goals between health care professionals and the person with diabetes, there may also be lack of agreement between health care professionals themselves, so that patients may receive conflicting advice depending on the health care professional they are consulting with. A recent survey of 152 health care professionals at 21 paediatric diabetes centres, asked respondents to indicate what the ideal HbA1c values for young people with type 1 diabetes should be (deBeaufort et al., 2006). The results showed that different professionals had different target values. The survey also showed that there was just as much variability within most diabetes centres as there was between them.

Good communication between health care professionals and the patient would seem to be an elusive goal for some, and assumptions that the doctor 'knows best' may remain commonly accepted. Fisher describes the work of doctors as both social and political in nature (Fisher, 1984). It is social in terms of the interaction that takes place between health care professional and patient, but also in terms of ideas about illness, the sick role (Parsons, 1951) and how people respond to symptoms. It is political because it 'helps to sustain and reproduces the status quo ... [and by] controlling access to the health care system and providing exemptions for those whose illness they legitimate, doctors help to maintain the existing social order' (Fisher, 1984, p. 5). Interactions between health care professionals and people with diabetes take place within this framework of commonly held beliefs that the doctor is the 'expert' and the person with diabetes needs to carry out the advice given to him/her in order to optimize health and well-being.

Conclusions

Diabetes is one of the most common long-term conditions facing health care services this century. The implications for nursing are wide ranging, including how best to work with both other health care professionals and the person with diabetes to support appropriate self-management of the condition. Ideas about health and illness, issues around communication and the relationship between health care professionals and patients are fundamental considerations of current health care policy and nursing practice for diabetes. An empowerment approach to care, actively encouraged as the ideal approach to diabetes care in current policy, remains to be fully implemented into practice.

References

Anderson R.J., K.E. Freedland, R.E. Clouse and P.J. Lustman, 'The prevalence of comorbid depression in adults with diabetes: a meta-analysis', *Diabetes Care*, 24: 6 (2001) 1069–1078.

Anderson R.M. and M.M. Funnell, *The Art of Empowerment* (Alexandria: American Diabetes Association, 2000).

Bandura A., 'Self-efficacy: toward a unifying theory of behaviour change', *Psychological Review*, 84 (1977) 191–215.

Banks D., *Living with Diabetes* (Milton Keynes: Open University, 2005).

Baradaran H., and R. Knill-Jones, 'Assessing knowledge, attitudes and understanding of type 2 diabetes amongst ethnic groups

I Glasgow, Scotland', *Practical Diabetes International*, 21: 4 (2004) 143–148.

Barlow J.H., and J. Sturt, 'Self-management interventions for people with chronic conditions in primary care: Examples from arthritis, asthma and diabetes', *Health Education Journal* 61: 4 (2002) 365–378.

Benner J.S., R.J. Glynn, H. Mogun, P.J. Neumann, M.C. Weinstein and J. Avorn, 'Long-term persistence in use of statin therapy in elderly patients', *Journal of the American Medical Association*, 288: 4 (2002) 455–461.

Chapman R.H., J.S. Benner, A.A. Petrilla, J.C. Tierce, S.R. Collins, D.S. Battleman and J.S. Schwartz, 'Predictors of adherence with antihypertensive and lipid-lowering therapy', *Archives of Internal Medicine*, 165: 10 (2005) 1147–1152.

Chowdhury T.A., and S.A. Lasker, 'Complications and cardiovascular risk factors in South Asian and Europeans with early onset type 2 diabetes', *QJM: An International Journal of Medicine,* 95: 4 (2002) 241–246.

Clark J.A., and E.G. Mishler, 'Attending to patients' stories: reframing the clinical task', *Sociology of Health & Illness*, 14: 3 (1992) 344–372.

Curtis S., J. Beirne and E. Jude, 'Advantages of training Asian diabetes support workers for Asian families and diabetes health care professionals', *Practical Diabetes International*, 20: 6 (2003) 215–218.

de Beaufort C., on behalf of the Hvidøre Study Group on Childhood Diabetes, 'Exploring and explaining center differences?', *Pediatric Diabetes*, 7: 5 (2006) 9.

Department of Health (DH), *National Service Framework for Diabetes* (London: Department of Health, 2001).

Department of Health (DH), *National Service Framework for Diabetes: Delivery strategy* (London: Department of Health, 2003).

Department of Health (DH), *Making Every Young Person with Diabetes Matter: Report of the Children and Young People with Diabetes Working Group* (London: Department of Health, 2007).

DESMOND Collaborative, *DESMOND Newly Diagnosed Module: Educator Manual*, 2nd edn (Leicester: DESMOND Collaborative, 2004).

DH Diabetes Policy Team, *Making Every Young Person with Diabetes Matter: Report of the Children and Young People with Diabetes Working Group* (London: Diabetes Policy Team, 2007).

Diabetes UK, *State of the Nations 2005: Progress Made in Delivering the National Diabetes Frameworks* (online) http://www.diabetes.nhs.

uk/downloads/StateOfNations.pdf [last accessed 5 December 2006].

Ferner R.E., 'Is concordance the primrose path to health?', *British Medical Journal*, 327 (2003) 821–822 .

Fisher S., 'Doctor-patient communication: a social and micropolitical performance', *Sociology of Health and Illness*, 6: 1 (1984) 1–29.

Greenhalgh T., C. Helman and A.M. Chowdhury, 'Health beliefs and folk models of diabetes in British Bangladeshis: a qualitative study', *British Medical Journal*, 316 (1998) 978–983.

Haynes R.B., X. Yao, A. Degani, S. Kripalani, A. Garg and H.P. McDonald, 'Interventions for enhancing medication adherence (Review)', *Cochrane Database of Systematic Reviews*, 2 (2007).

Hiscock J., R. Legard and D. Snape, *Listening to Diabetes Service Users: Qualitative Findings for the National Service Framework* (London: Department of Health, 2001).

Lerner B., 'From careless consumptives to recalcitrant patients: the historical construction of non-compliance', *Social Science and Medicine*, 45: 9 (1997)1423–1431.

Lloyd C.E., P.H. Dyer and A.H. Barnett, 'Prevalence of symptoms of depression and anxiety in a diabetes clinic population', *Diabetic Medicine*, 17 (2000) 198–202.

Lloyd C.E., S. Mughal, J. Sturt, P. O'Hare and A.H. Barnett, 'Using self-complete questionnaires in a South Asian population with diabetes: problems and solutions', *Diversity in Health & Social Care*, 3 (2006) 245–251.

Lorig K., D.S. Sobel, A.L. Stewart, B.W. Brown, A. Barndura and P. Ritter et al., 'Evidence suggesting that a chronic disease self-management programme can improve health status whilst reducing hospitalization: A randomised trial', *Medical Care*, 37 (1999) 5–14.

Lustman P.J., L.S. Griffith and R.E. Clouse, 'Recognising and managing depression in patients with diabetes', in R.R. Rubin and B.J. Anderson (eds), *Practical Psychology for Diabetes Clinicians* (Alexandria: American Diabetes Association 1996).

Lustman P.J., L.S. Griffith, K.E. Freedland, S.S. Kissel and R.E. Clouse, 'Cognitive behaviour therapy for depression in type 2 diabetes mellitus. A randomized controlled trial', *Annals of Internal Medicine*, 129: 8 (1998) 613–621.

May C., G. Allison, A. Chapple, C. Chew-Graham, C. Dixon, L. Gask, R. Graham, A. Rogers and M. Roland, 'Framing the doctor-patient relationship in chronic illness: a comparative study of general practitioners' accounts', *Sociology of Health & Illness*, 26: 2 (2004) 135–158.

National Diabetes Support Team, *The Psychological Impact of Diabetes* (online) http://www.diabetes.nhs.uk/Reading_room/ Factsheets.asp [last accessed 5 December 2006].

NICE, *Guidance on the Use of Patient-Education Models for Diabetes. Technology Appraisal 60* (London: NICE, 2003).

NICE, CG023 Depression (amended): management of depression in primary and secondary care (London: NICE, 2007). Available from www.nice.org.uk/GG023. Reproduced with permission.

Page P., D.G. Verstraete, J.R. Robb and D.D. Etzwiler, 'Patient recall of self-care recommendations in diabetes', *Diabetes Care*, 4 (1981) 96–98.

Parkin T., and T.C. Skinner, 'Discrepancies between patient and professionals recall and perception of an outpatient consultation', *Diabetic Medicine*, 20: 11 (2003) 909–914.

Parkin T., K. Barnard, S. Cradock, P. Pettman and T.C. Skinner, 'Does professional centred training improve consultation outcomes?', *Practical Diabetes International*, 23: 6 (2006) 253–256.

Parsons T., *The Social System* (London: Routledge and Kegan Paul, 1951).

Sabate E., *Adherence to Long-Term Therapies: Evidence for Action* (Geneva: World Health Organization, 2003) http://www.who. int/topics/patient_adherence/en/ [last accessed 10 September 2007].

Skinner T.C., K. Barnard, S. Cradock and T. Parkin, 'Patient and professional accuracy of recalled treatment decisions in out-patient consultations', *Diabetic Medicine*, 24: 5 (2007) 557–560.

Simpson S.H., D.T. Eurich, S.R. Majumdar, R.S. Padwal, R.T. Tsuyuki, J. Varney and J.S. Johnson, 'A meta-analysis of the association between adherence to drug therapy and mortality', *British Medical Journal*, 333: 15 (2006) EPub: BMJ, doi:10.1136/ bmj.38875.675486.55 (published 21 June 2006).

Tindall W.N., R.S. Beardsley and C.L. Kimberlin (eds), *Communication Skills in Pharmacy Practice: a Practical Guide for Students and Practitioners* (Philadelphia, PA: Lippincott, Willliams and Wilkins, 2001).

Toobert D.J., S.E. Hampson and R.E. Glasgow, 'The summary of diabetes self-care activities measure: results from seven studies and a revised scale', *Diabetes Care*, 23 (2000) 943–950.

Vermeire E., J. Wens, P. Van Royen, Y. Biot, H. Hearnshaw and A. Lindenmeyer, 'Interventions for improving adherence to treatment recommendations in people with type 2 Diabetes Mellitus', *Cochrane Database of Systematic Reviews*, 2005, 2. Art. No.: CD003638. DOI: 10.1002/14651858.CD003638.pub2.

Vyas A., A.Z. Haidery, P.G. Wiles, S. Gill, C. Roberts and J.K. Cruickshank, 'A pilot randomized trial in primary care to investigate and improve knowledge, awareness and self-management among South Asians with diabetes in Manchester', *Diabetic Medicine*, 20 (2003)1022–1026.

Woodcock A., and A.L. Kinmonth, 'Patient concerns in their first year with type 2 diabetes: patient and practice nurse views', *Patient Education Counseling*, 42 (2001) 257–270.

The X-Pert Programme, http://www.xpert-diabetes.org.uk/ (last accessed 15 September 2008).

7 'Getting to know myself': changing needs and gaining knowledge among people with cancer

Jonathan Tritter

Introduction

Being diagnosed with cancer is no longer the death sentence it once was and cancer as a topic is no longer taboo. Yet the World Health Organization's Cancer Research Agency estimate that, there were 3.2 million new cases of cancer in 2006 and 1.7 million deaths from the disease in the whole of Europe (Ferlay et al., 2007). Further it has been estimated that up to 30 per cent of all individuals in the developed world will present clinically with one of a wide variety of cancers at some time in their lives (WCRF/AICR, 1997, p. 55). In the United Kingdom, more than 276,000 people were diagnosed with cancer in 2003 and more than 153,000 people died from cancer in 2004 (Cancer Research UK, 2006). Thus, the impact of cancer on all of our lives is great, whether directly or indirectly.

This chapter reports some findings of recent research into patients' understanding and perceptions of their disease. In particular it focuses on how cancer patients define their own needs for support and self management and act in order to satisfy them. Thus, while acknowledging the importance of the delivery of care and clinical issues it is the types, timing and sources of support, using as broad a definition as possible of these concepts which is the central focus of this study.

There have been significant improvements in the medical diagnosis and treatment of cancer and almost a half of cancers are now 'cured' (Tubiana, 1992). The medical understanding of cancer has increased dramatically and while still highly contested, the concept of cure remains primarily defined in relation to five year survival. But far less research has been conducted on patients' understandings of their illness or on their reactions to the various medical interventions intended to cure them.

For patients the nature of the disease and its treatment results in periods when they feel perfectly normal. 'I think that is one of the most bizarre things about cancer, I'm a real example of it. But you are so basically fit, I felt absolutely great, and you think, you've got somebody else, because I feel so great, you feel fine actually' (Roy, Bristol).

Their treatment, however, can often mean significant discomfort and illness and may require repeated interventions. Therefore, in some ways cancer can be best understood as both a chronic and acute illness. Further, cancer treatment typically involves primary, acute and community based health care and involves the integrated delivery of multiple medical specialities. Finally, cancer and its treatment is high profile in both medical and media terms.

The organization and delivery of cancer care through the British National Health Service has undergone significant change following the modernization led by the NHS Cancer Plan (DH, 2000a). These shifts are a product of a report by the Expert Advisory Group on Cancer to the Chief Medical Officers of England and Wales (Calman and Hine, 1995) on guidance to purchasers and providers of cancer services. Yet the majority of decisions made for, or on behalf of, cancer patients are done so by health professionals with little input from patients (Degner et al., 1997), despite many doctors believing that patients have sufficient involvement and information (Calkins et al., 1997). In addition there continue to be inequities in treatment for instance both men with prostate cancer and patients in London experiencing significantly worse care than patients in other parts of the country (National Audit Office, 2005).

The proposed changes in the delivery of cancer care are based on a public service medical context which increasingly acknowledges the importance of patients' views and involvement in their treatment (DH, 2000b, 2003, 2004). In Britain, beginning in the 1990s there has been a consistent call for increased patient participation in the evaluation and planning of health care beginning with the publication of Local Voices (NHSME, 1992) and Consumers and Research in the NHS (DH, 1995) but carried through legislation in 2001 and 2003. Currently new legislation before parliament will radically change the structures and powers that underpin opportunities for local people to engage with the evaluation and development of health services (DH, 2006a, b) as well as the current stress on patient satisfaction and consumer audit.

Yet the vast majority of patient involvement within the NHS is based on problematic patient satisfaction surveys, 'citizen juries' or token patient representation on consultative groups (Baggott, 2005; Rigge, 1995). Typically patients are seen as having a limited, and usually passive, role in decision-making and treating their illness. There are, however, exceptions where providers, patients and purchasers work together to define the best cancer care (Millar, 1996) and research (Bradburn et al., 1995). Further evidence and tools to support best practice in patient and public involvement in service development are available from the NHS Centre for Involvement (http://www.nhscentreforinvolvement.nhs.uk) and in research from INVOLVE (http://www.involve.org.uk, last accessed 15 September 2008). Similarly there is clear evidence that when patients and health care professional are jointly involved in decision making the efficacy of the treatment and patient compliance increases (Blanchard et al., 1990; Cassileth et al., 1980; Fitzpatrick and Hopkins, 1981; Locker and Dunt, 1978; Wooley et al., 1978).

For many people after diagnosis and initial treatment for cancer the primary issue becomes how they live with their condition. For some commentators, particularly in the United States, cancer is considered a 'chronic illness' (Department of Health and Human Services, 2007), while others reject this while affirming the long term nature of the condition and its consequences (Tritter and Calnan, 2002). Recurrence of the disease can happen years after initial treatment has been concluded compromizing the relevance of 'cure' as a concept and leading many people with a sense of abiding insecurity about the future. Treatment for cancer, therefore, can be conceptualized as acute treatment episodes with long latent periods with little or no direct medical intervention where the situation is primarily based on self-management (Holman and Lorig, 2000).

Research methods

This research was designed to explore cancer patients' needs for support and self-management. Three types of primary data were collected based on a two-stage focus-group and a brief questionnaire. The data was collected between August 1997 and July 1998 from 54 cancer patients during eight focus group meetings in metropolitan areas of England. Each group lasted between 90 minutes and three hours and was hosted in an informal environment in either a house or a hotel. The quantitative data from the short pre-meeting questionnaire provides details of basic demographic information as well as an outline of the patient's pathway or 'Cancer Journey' including their type of cancer, date of diagnosis and treatment regime.

Simple analysis of the questionnaire data applying descriptive statistics was carried out using Statistical Package for the Social Sciences (SPSS). The focus groups were all recorded and transcribed verbatim. The transcriptions were analyzed using ATLAS.ti, a computer package designed to aid textual interpretation. The systematic coding of the transcripts was based on a series of meetings involving the entire steering group and multiple-coding of the same piece of text together with our comments on the process provided the necessary complexity. Thus we adopted a grounded theory approach to our analysis (Glaser and Strauss, 1967), using 'constant comparative analysis, development of theoretical concepts and statements, and theoretical sampling as well as the usual supporting techniques of theoretical coding and memoing' (Strauss and Corbin, 1997, pp. 1–2). Our conceptualization was aided by a 'debriefing' meeting between the three researchers who collected the qualitative data discussions following each focus group, but was a product of the entire steering group.

The construction of the focus groups in the study

The focus groups were divided into two specific sections with the second stage being covered in a second meeting the following evening. This ensured that the participants had sufficient time for discussion and had built up sufficient empathy with other members of the group to feel comfortable discussing sensitive topics. The first meeting aimed to introduce participants to one another and identify the varied needs that patients' had experienced during their 'Cancer Journey'. The second meeting began with a report back to the group summarizing the key points of discussion from the previous evening. Then using a diagram of the Cancer Journey and a list of potential sources of support and assistance we asked participants to identify the point at which a particular need, or set of needs, was greatest. Patients were then asked to explain how they had met this need and who had been involved. Finally, we asked the participants to suggest who, ideally, should provide for a particular need and when and how this should be provided.

The research sample

Participants were recruited in four metropolitan areas: Bath, Bristol, London and Manchester. In each region we convened two different focus groups. Recruitment was based on a combination of clinical settings and the voluntary sector with a minimum of three different sources being used in each area. In each recruitment setting information sheets with an attached questionnaire were displayed in a waiting area and interested patients could complete them and return them to a collection point. This process resulted in a diverse participant population who were relatively unfamiliar with each other but include people with a range of cancers and who had been treated in a variety of different settings. As the recruitment was in part through specialist cancer clinics we were required to obtain approval from four separate medical research ethic committees. Table 7.1 provides details of the numbers of participants and locations of the focus groups convened.

Table 7.1 Demographic and disease related characteristics of the sample

Number of patients in the study		54
Number of focus groups		8
Age range		30–77 years
Mean age		54 years
Gender	Female	40
	Male	14
Location	Bath	15
	Bristol	13
	London	15
	Manchester	11
Cancer Type (primary)	Breast	27
	Gastrointestinal	8
	Gynaecological	4
	Lymphoma	5
	Melanoma	3
	Leukaemia	3
	Other (one each)	4
Time out of treatment	Range	0–362 months
	Mean	35 months

As with any study based on a self-selected sample it is likely there is a bias towards those who hold stronger views or who tend to be more active. There are clearly categories of patients who did not participate. Thus the sample has twice as many women as men and very few ethnic minority participants. However, drawing from a range of voluntary and clinical settings did not allow us to target specific patient population but did serve to maximize the variation in our sample and ensured that the research was based on the full spectrum of patient types and a wide range of experience. In all patients had been treated in 31 different hospitals and while the majority had primary breast cancer 19 distinct types of cancer were apparent in our sample.

Patients were keen to participate and share their knowledge, experience and understanding within a research framework that preserved their views and was not dominated by prescribed theoretical and service-delivery issues that tends to typify research that involves patients.

Time, experience and understanding

Peoples' reactions to cancer are a product of their understanding of cancer and their conception of themselves as a 'cancer patient'. Different reactions and lifestyles require different needs. This research aims to begin to map patients' needs on to the position in their treatment career or 'Cancer Journey'. The latter is a term defined by the National Cancer Alliance (1995) and has a clear relationship to what Wiener et al. (1997) have termed a *trajectory*. But to do this requires the mapping of both the biomedically defined Cancer Journey and a parallel but distinct moral career. For as patients' understanding of cancer changes so does their reaction to their situation, their life-style and their needs.

In Britain the route from initial concern through investigation, diagnosis, treatment and 'cure' or cessation of treatment is a convoluted one involving multiple sites, specialists and treatments. The first stage involves an initial referral for specialist investigation by a General Practitioner or as a result of a screening process. The investigation, typically in a hospital setting, may involve a range of tests and examinations with the results often unconfirmed for several weeks.

> I think one of the worst things is the wait for the diagnosis. You have the mammograms and biopsies and it's that awful period of waiting. And of course the power of the mind is so great and even though you know in your mind that it's cancer, it's got to be said. (Penny, Bristol)

Following the confirmation of the diagnosis patients are again referred to a cancer specialist with whom discussions and decisions about treatment are made. Typically, three types of treatment are seen as biomedically most appropriate for cancer: chemotherapy, radiotherapy and surgery. Patients may have one or more of these treatments and the order, intensity and duration vary. Furthermore, some treatments are undertaken for palliative rather than curative reasons. Often the choice of treatment is heavily dependent on who the patient is first referred to. As one patient understood it, 'I did feel that I happened to be in the hospital at the wrong time. Because, the radiology department grabbed me and radiated me and if the other department had got me I would have had chemotherapy. I'm quite convinced of that' (Roy, Bristol).

Following the patient's particular course of treatment they enter a monitoring phase which involved attending an outpatient clinic at set regular intervals for a 'check up'. Initially these visits are fairly frequent, fortnightly or monthly, but the gaps become larger and are eventually every six months or a year. Monitoring is presented as providing an opportunity for the early identification of secondary cancer but in practice there is so little continuity in the medical personnel who see a particular patient that there is little chance of such detection.

> I'd finished my radiation treatment and a couple of doctors had a prod at me and a couple of trainee doctors. So it was great, fine, wonderful and then this very quiet doctor in radiology, came in and prodded me and said 'you're off again'. And he found it (a secondary tumour) straight away. Nobody else had found it. About six of them had missed it. (Roy, Bristol)

There is evidence from Canadian and European studies (Brada, 1995; Grunfeld et al., 1996; Holli and Hakama, 1989) that follow-up monitoring is less effective at identifying early onset of secondaries than 'spontaneous' patient-led visits though it is often very important to patients. After five years of monitoring with no recurrence of cancer patients are said to be 'clear' or in remission.

For some patients there is no medical treatment available that will 'cure' the cancer. This may be due to the type of cancer or to its stage of advancement. Patients in this situation may be offered treatment for palliative rather than curative reasons. Palliative care, pain relief and hospice services may also be made available to patients at this stage of their journey.

The Cancer Journey can be likened to a train journey. There are a series of stations where not all trains will stop and junctions that permit different pathways and iterations of the stages in the Cancer Journey. Each station offers an opportunity for leaving or changing trains. In this sense it is the stations on the Cancer Journey that provide points at which shifts in individuals' understanding and self-definition as cancer patients may take place. These shifts form an epistemological journey in which patients make sense of their cancer

and act on the basis of their understanding even if it is sometimes at odds with accepted biomedical advice. The epistemological or identity journey of a cancer patient can be likened to
what Goffman (1961) referred to as the 'moral career' of the
mental patient:

> The moral career of a person of a given social category involves
> a standard sequence of changes in his [sic] way of conceiving of
> selves, including importantly his own. These half-buried lines of
> development can be followed by studying his moral experiences-
> that is, happenings which mark a turning point in the way in which
> the person views the world-although the particularities of their view
> may be difficult to establish. (Goffman, 1961, p. 168)

For patients, their reaction to having cancer and their identity
as an individual diagnosed with cancer is dependent on their
understanding and definition of their cancer. As one patient
suggested 'I firmly believe that I can't control my cancer, I
equally firmly believe that I can control how I handle it.' (Sue,
London 2, 1). But their understanding of their cancer changes
as a product of both their experiences of treatment and over
time and it is the 'stories' that they told us in the focus groups
that demonstrate how they made sense of their lives (Mathieson
and Stam, 1995). As Goffman suggests: 'The concept of career,
then, allows one to move back and forth between the personal
and the public, between the self and its significant society.'
(Goffman, 1961, p. 127). Despite the multiple sources of variation I want to suggest that there are particular points in the
Cancer Journey that often are associated with shifts in patients'
epistemological journeys or moral careers. It is at these points
that patients adjust their identities and these shifts are reflected
in changed behaviour to which I now turn (see Figure 7.1).

Diagnosis

The vast majority of patients react to a diagnosis of cancer with
a frenzy of information seeking activities.

> I read feverishly for about a month afterwards, anything I could
> get my hands on, I've read all the pamphlets, and then I read this

research paper on meningeoma and then that sort of phase stopped and I decided not to read anymore

Facilitator: Why?

Because I felt I had sufficient information really and it was getting a bit silly and obsessive, that was just for me. (Martin, London)

This is, to an extent an admission of ignorance and seeking a personal definition of cancer, their particular cancer and what a cancer patient is. This is the first station on the epistemological Cancer Journey. But, as time passes and patients are processed and progress along the 'Cancer Journey', most come to a different understanding of their cancer and condition and their information seeking decreases. But the definition of cancer that they have arrived at, results in a change in behaviour and a shift in the needs that they express.

For some patients their understanding of cancer is that it is a disease that is amenable to medical treatment. They trust in the medical profession and believe in curative interventions. The epistemological journey for these patients deviates very little from the biomedical Cancer Journey. They do not wish to know more about their cancer or their treatment and do not seek to participate in decisions about their care instead leaving everything to healthcare professionals. In some sense, these patients ignore their illness and try to act 'normally'.

I thought, I've been told what it is. I don't want to know all the ins and outs. I just want to know, can they cure it. So I just didn't want to read lots and lots and it's like during the time I had breast cancer, there seemed to be something on the radio or television all last year about breast cancer. Normally I would watch these programs with avid interest. But, I didn't want to know while I was going through it. (Jackie, Bristol)

For others, also a minority, being diagnosed with cancer is clearly a death sentence and if this particular 'episode' is not mortal then secondary cancer is sure to follow soon after. As one patient put it 'It's always there, when I was very depressed I wanted it to hurry up and get me so that the waiting was like waiting for someone to come and chop your head off if you like.' (Pam, Manchester). The meaning of the diagnosis of cancer for these patients leads to a clear sense of proximate

mortality and a truncated life and a different range of behavioural responses.

Monitoring

For most patients their reaction to the move to 'monitoring' following their treatment is very mixed. While they are
relieved that often very uncomfortable and distressing interventions are at an end they also express a sense of concern and
isolation associated with moving out of a clinical setting. They
are no longer the focus of attention, on a frequent basis, by
health care professionals who they see as responsible for curing
their cancer.

> At the end, when you have done your treatment, it's a funny thing,
> but I felt abandoned. When they said don't come back for a year, I
> thought, 'My goodness, that's a long time.' I felt really abandoned.
> (Frances, Bath)
>
> Every single day...and you see the nurse for the last time. You have
> that last 'Oh yes, you seem all right, bye-bye.' And you walk out of
> there and you think, 'Gosh, I'm on my own now.' ... The feeling is like
> when you leave school when you are 16 or 18. (Rob, Bristol)

Their identity as cancer patient is more difficult to define without repeated visits and references to clinical settings. This often
leads to patients pursuing a regime aimed at getting them 'fit'
which may include an array of complementary or alternative
therapies. There is an inevitable tension in a self-definition as a
cancer patient but one who is no longer being treated for their
cancer. A new identity and definition of cancer patient must be
constructed that is less dependent on 'treatment'.

Diagnosis of secondary cancer

For most patients who are diagnosed with secondary cancer
this is far more shocking than their initial diagnosis:

> I am right at the end now between secondaries and no further med-
> ical treatment.... I was terrified for the first couple of days, especially

> when I thought I could be dead in 6 months, ... there is nothing to take into account the time between now and when we die, which is a place, that's a thing I didn't experience until 5 weeks ago, and that is really where you are in no mans land, so you can say the worse thing is when you were first diagnosed but for me the worst was getting secondaries. (Linda, London)

This second diagnosis provides evidence of the absence of curative biomedical intervention and raises the question of the potential impossibility of cure. Thus, the definition of cancer patient, as an individual being treated for cancer and on the way to recovery is no longer possible to maintain: 'I thought well, my mother's 81 this year and I thought to myself I'll never be 80. I know I won't, it's just this feeling. So, I'm not an optimistic person. I just get on with it' (Frances, Bath).

For some patients, the immediacy of personal mortality provides a spur to action. All of the activities previously being postponed until later, or after retirement, are embarked upon:

> I used to be always spending my money on the home or my daughter, and saying I'd love to go to Egypt but I can't afford it. Now I go and have the holidays that I want to have and I do all the things that I want to do which somehow I didn't have the time to do before. (Caroline, Bristol)

Whatever the reaction patients in this situation speak of seeing the world differently – of periods of heightened experience:

> I've got time to pursue things that are right for me and to a certain extent there is a guilt around that and I think you have to get over all of that, but also looking at that tree down there, I'm sure that, in a sense has changed.
> *Facilitator*: You wouldn't have seen the tree?
> I would have seen the tree but I may not have seen it in the same sort of way, I don't think necessarily that is about me going through cancer, I think it's more to do with having more time to appreciate the things around me and that is about mortality. (Martin, London)

Thus, patients at this point are once again changing their identity to incorporate the now more clearly truncated lifespan they expect. This has consequences for how they decide to spend the time remaining and who they choose to spend it with.

For many patients this change provides a license to act in ways that go against social expectations. In some sense they may feel that they are now going to be far more active in choosing to do things that they like and unwilling to put up with those they do not:

> I had a friend for ten years and she was always making barbed remarks which really irritated. And I would really have liked to have told her I don't want anything to do with you. But I didn't and I tolerated her for ten years. And when I came out of hospital after radiotherapy, she rang me up the day after I came out. And she said 'Oh, hello. Was it really terrible for you in the hospital? Was it really awful for you?' And I said 'I'm so glad you rang because there's something I really want to say to you.' And she said 'Oh yes, go on, you first.' And I said 'Okay, I don't want anything else to do with you. I've never liked you and please don't ring me up again.' And she said 'Well, get it off your chest.' And I said, 'I just have.' (Libby, Bristol)

In less drastic examples participants explained that they were changing their life to make it less stressful and complicated. Typically people with cancer sought to refocus their lives only on things they wanted to do and being with people they wanted to spend time with.

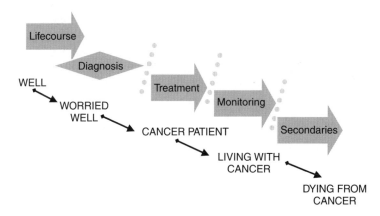

Figure 7.1 The moral career

Epistemological stages

What I have illustrated in this chapter is a series of identities that cancer patients adopt in response to their changing definition of cancer and self. These shifts are a production of multiple factors though chiefly experience of treatment, information and time. What is suggested is not a series of coping mechanisms, or shallow adaptations designed to allow patients to continue to survive, but rather a series of transformed identities based on particular understandings of cancer and what it is to be a cancer patient. Thus, the model of self-identity being suggested is dynamic rather that the static series of psychological stances proposed by some commentators (Greer, 1991; Greer et al., 1979; Greer and Watson, 1987). It is a model that owes much to the work of Mathieson and Stam (1995). They suggest that:

> A patient who lives with cancer finds herself in a nexus of dynamic psychosocial events. These events often result in reports of loss or productive functioning, financial strain, family stress, personal distress, stigma, and threats to former self images. Taken together, these events signal that one's identity will forcibly undergo transformation. (Mathieson and Stam, 1995, p. 287)

Greer (1991) suggests five global categorical psychological stances: Denial (positive avoidance), Fighting spirit, Stoic acceptance (fatalism), Helplessness/hopelessness and Anxious pre-occupation that characterize patient reactions to cancer. I am suggesting instead, that patients are not fixed in particular categories but instead move between them as a product of their knowledge and experience. Further, that these movements are not random but clearly related to particular points on the Cancer Journey. Finally, that patient's needs are an expression of the particular identity they have constructed as a cancer patient.

Conclusions

The findings of this research emphasize the need to understand the patterned variation in patients' knowledge and understanding of their cancer and identity as cancer patients.

A key issue for all people with cancer is the sense of suddenly only having a limited time. For this sample of people with cancer this felt truncation of life led to a desire for speed in the diagnosis and treatment of their illness but had other significant impacts on how people understood their cancer and lived their life as a cancer patient differently from the way they had prior to diagnosis. Nurses and in particular specialist cancer nurses increasingly have a role to play in ensuring that people with cancer and their families are informed about the nature of their situation and the options available to them. The increased emphasis on patient experience in cancer services and throughout healthcare more broadly has particular resonance for the caring role of nurses and the ways they often serve as translators between medics and patients.

These shifts in identity are structured and related to particular points on the biomedically defined Cancer Journey. What people with cancer need, and when this should be provided needs to be considered in relation to their identity. For example, the offer and take up of counselling or an 'information prescription' (see http://www.informationprescription.info, last accessed 15 September 2008) must be considered in relation to people's identify journey. The need for information is often felt intensely at the point of diagnosis and then further information about side-effects of treatment. Later in the cancer journey, when the person with cancer is being monitored a different type of information, perhaps relating to healthy living is likely to be far more appropriate. Similarly, counselling or other supportive intervention need to be considered in relation to the kinds of needs most likely to emerge at different points in the identify journey. A clearer view of the nature of patient understanding permits more effective and appropriate clinical and non-clinical interventions that will be suitable to the identity that particular cancer patients create.

It is clear from this research that patients attempt to make sense of the world, a world that is changed by the diagnosis and treatment of their cancer. That the way people seek, incorporate and act based on a particular understanding of cancer is for them rational even if it differs from traditional biomedical views. Patients' reactions are not coping mechanisms but reflections of a transformed identity; an identity which is based on a particularistic understanding of cancer and what it is to be a cancer patient. Patient-centred care must take in to account the changing identify of the patient in order to ensure the best possible care, compliance and outcomes.

References

Baggott R., 'A funny thing happened on the way to the forum', *Public Administration*, 83 (2005), 533–551.

Blanchard C., M. Labrecque, J. Ruckdeschel and E. Blanchard, 'Physician behaviors, patient perceptions, and patient characteristics as predictors of satisfaction of hospitalized adult cancer patients', *Cancer*, 65 (1990) 186–190.

Brada M., 'Is there a need to follow-up cancer patients?', *European Journal of Cancer*, 31A (1995) 655–657.

Bradburn J., J. Maher, R. Adewuyi-Dalton, E. Grunfeld, T. Lancaster and D. Mant, 'Developing clinical trial protocols: The use of patient focus groups', *Psycho-Oncology*, 4 (1995) 107–112.

Calkins D., R. Davis, P. Reiley, R. Phillips, K. Pineo, T. Delbanco and L. Iezzoni, 'Patient-physician communication at hospital discharge and patients' understanding of the postdischarge treatment plan', *Archives of Internal Medicine*, 157 (1997), 1026–1030.

Calman K., and D. Hine, *A Policy Framework for Commissioning Cancer Services; A Report of the Expert Advisory Group on Cancer to the Chief Medical Officers of England and Wales* (London: Department of Health and Welsh Office, 1995).

Cancer Research UK, *Cancer Statistics* (London: Cancer Research UK, 2006) *http://cancerresearchuk.org/cancerstats* (last accessed 16 April 2007).

Cassileth B., R. Zupkis, K. Sutton-Smith and V. March, 'Information and participation preferences among cancer patients', *Annals of Internal Medicine*, 92 (1980) 832–836.

Degner L.F., L.J. Kristajanson, D. Bowman, J.A. Sloan, K.C. Carriere, J. O'Neil, B. Bilodeau, P. Watson and B. Mueller, 'Information needs and decisional preferences in women with breast cancer', *Journal of the American Medical Association*, 277 (1997) 1485–1492.

Department of Health (DH), *Building on the Best: Choice, Responsiveness and Equity in the NHS* (Cm 6079) (London: HMSO, 2003).

Department of Health (DH), *Consumers and Research in the NHS* (Leeds: National Health Service Executive, 1995).

Department of Health (DH), *The NHS Cancer Plan: A Plan for Investment , a Plan for Reform* (London: Department of Health, 2000a).

Department of Health (DH), *The NHS Plan* (Cm 4818–I), (London: Department of Health, 2000b).

Department of Health (DH), *NHS Improvement Plan*, (Leeds: Department of Health, 2004).

Department of Health (DH), *Government Response to Whom it May Concern: 'A Stronger Local Voice'* (London: Department of Health, 2006a).

Department of Health (DH), *A Stronger Local Voice in the Development of Health and Social Care Services* (London: Department of Health, 2006b).

Department of Health and Human Services, *National Center for Health Statistics* (Hyatsville, MD: National Center for Health Statistics, 2007) *http://www.cdc.gov/nchs/datawh/nchsdefs/health condition.htm#chronic* (last accessed 16 April 2007).

Ferlay J., P. Autier, M. Boniol, M. Heanue, M. Colombet and P. Boyle, 'Estimates of cancer incidence an mortality in Europe in 2006', *Annals of Oncology*, 18 (2007) 581–592.

Fitzpatrick R., and D. Hopkins, 'Patients' satisfaction with communication in neurological outpatient clinics', *Journal of Psychosomatic Research*, 25 (1981) 329–334.

Glaser B., and A. Strauss, *The Discovery of Grounded Theory* (Chicago: Aldine, 1967).

Goffman E., *Asylums: Essays on the Social Situation of Mental Patients and other Inmates* (Chicago: Aldine, 1961).

Greer S., 'Psychological response to cancer and survival', *Psychological Medicine*, 21 (1991) 43–49.

Greer S., and M. Watson, 'Mental adjustment to cancer: Its measurement and prognostic importance', *Cancer Surveys*, 6 (1987) 439–453.

Greer S., T. Morris and K. Pettingale, 'Psychological response to breast cancer: Effect on outcome', *Lancet*, ii (1979) 785–787.

Grunfeld E., D. Mant, P. Yudkin, R. Adewuyi-Dalton, D. Cole, J. Stewart, R. Fitzpatrick and M. Vessey, 'Routine follow up of breast cancer in primary care: randomised trial', *British Medical Journal*, 313 (1996) 665–669.

Holli K., and M. Hakama, 'Treatment of the terminal stages of breast cancer', *British Medical Journal*, 298 (1989) 13–14.

Holman H. and K. Lorig, 'Patients as partners in managing chronic disease', *British Medical Journal*, 320 (2000) 526–527.

Locker D., and D. Dunt, 'Theoretical and methodological issues in sociological studies of consumer satisfaction with medical care', *Social Science and Medicine*, 12 (1978) 283–292.

Mathieson C., and H. Stam, 'Renegotiating identity: cancer narratives', *Sociology of Health & Illness*, 17: 3 (1995) 283–306.

Millar B., 'Cultural revolution', *Health Service Journal*, 106 (1996) 7.

National Audit Office, *Tackling Cancer: Improving the Patient Journey* (London: National Audit Office, 2005).

National Cancer Alliance, *Directory of Cancer Specialists* (Oxford: National Cancer Alliance, 1995).

National Health Service Management Executive (NHSME), *Local Voices* (London: Department of Health, 1992).

Rigge M., 'Does public opinion matter? (Yes/No/Don't know)', *Health Service Journal*, 105 (1995) 26–27.

Strauss A., and J. Corbin, (eds), *Grounded Theory in Practice* (London: Sage, 1997).

Tritter J., and M. Calnan, 'Cancer as a chronic illness? Reconsidering categorization and exploring experience', researching users' experiences of health care: The case of cancer', *Special Issue of European Journal of Cancer Care*, 11 (2002) 161–165.

Tubiana M., 'The role of local treatment in the cure of cancer', *European Journal of Cancer and Clinical Oncology*, 28a 12 (1992) 2061–2069.

Wiener C., A. Strauss, S. Fagerhaugh and B. Suczek, 'Trajectories, biographies, and the evolving medical technology scene', in A. Strauss and J. Corbin (eds), *Grounded Theory in Practice* (London: Sage, 1997).

Wooley F., R. Kane, C. Hughes and D. Wright, 'The effects of doctor patient communication on satisfaction and outcome of care', *Social Science and Medicine*, 12 (1978) 123–128.

World Cancer Research Fund/American Institute for Cancer Research (WCRF/AICR), *Food, Nutrition and the Prevention of Cancer: A Global Perspective* (Washington, DC: WCRF/AICR, 1997).

8 HIV/AIDS: a highly stigmatized long term condition

Erica Richardson

Introduction

There are now a number of communicable diseases which, with appropriate treatment, may be framed as long term conditions. However, as a new communicable disease which is treatable but incurable and one which is predominantly sexually transmitted, HIV/AIDS and those living with the virus are feared and highly stigmatized. The experience of living with HIV/AIDS has been used to explore many of the issues common to the sociology of all long term conditions. Indeed, it has been argued that HIV/AIDS has received a disproportionate level of attention given that other conditions and illnesses are much more common (Kelly and Field, 1996). HIV/AIDS has been used to explore issues such as stigmatization and construction of the 'other' (Lupton, 1999; Sontag, 1991; Waldby, 1996); as well as biographical disruption and identity (Anderson and Doyal, 2004; Carricaburu and Pierret, 1995; Ciambrone, 2001). However, the exploration of these issues also underlines the aspect of HIV/AIDS which makes it so different to the other long term conditions covered in this book – People Living with HIV/AIDS (PLWHA) can pass the virus (and so the condition) to others in society.

In this chapter, the sociology of HIV/AIDS is explored from the patient perspective, concentrating on HIV infection as a lived experience rather than an epidemiological or clinical issue. First, the changing nature of HIV/AIDS is explained historically in terms of the developments in treatment options for PLWHA; current service provisions for PLWHA in the

United Kingdom; and the significance of the shifting definition of 'AIDS' as the 'final' stage of disease progression. In the second section, drawing on studies of HIV/AIDS in the United Kingdom and elsewhere, the stigma of HIV/AIDS is explored, focusing on how the infection came to be so highly stigmatized and the effect this has on the experience of living with HIV/AIDS. The continuing significance of stigmatization is then demonstrated through an analysis of recent events in the United Kingdom and the criminalization of 'reckless' HIV transmission. The chapter then concludes with a review of the key messages for practitioners, educators, researchers and policy makers; because in order to ensure holistic care for PLWHA it is necessary to understand how HIV has been stigmatized and what this means in practice.

The changing nature of HIV/AIDS: treatment, care, definitions

Developments in antiretroviral therapies

Through advances in antiretroviral therapies, HIV/AIDS in the developed world has now shifted from being a terminal to a chronic infection. Effective antiretroviral agents have been available since 1987, although early treatments were unsustainable or provided only partially effective outcomes. From 1996 more effective multi-drug therapies have been available and, currently, the most effective treatment for HIV is Highly Active Antiretroviral Therapy (HAART) – a combined drug regime which inhibits viral replication to the extent that viral drug resistance is smothered; although the combination is a delicate balancing act to avoid drug resistance, which would otherwise occur within weeks (Lange, 2006). The development of new agents, and consequent improvements in the treatment of HIV, have had a dramatic impact on HIV-related morbidity and mortality, but antiretrovirals are still a treatment and not a cure. Living with HIV is a lifelong condition which requires constant medication under close medical supervision. Consequently, HIV/AIDS remains a considerable cause of mortality in poorer countries because the cost of antiretrovirals is prohibitive for most PLWHA. National and global policy initiatives have therefore focused on broadening access to treatment by negotiating with the pharmaceutical industry to procure more affordable medicines while respecting international trade and property rights regulations (see Fleet and N'Daw, 2006; WHO, UNAIDS and UNICEF, 2007).

The main medical challenges of antiretroviral therapy are those of adherence and toxicity. Adherence is difficult because different pills need to be taken at different times throughout the day, everyday, either with or without food. Adherence to drug regimes varies depending on the type of drug being prescribed, the length of time for which it should be taken and the complexity of the drug regimen, that is, it depends on the social context in which illness and treatment are experienced rather than on the characteristics of individual patients. For HAART, negotiating the stigma of HIV/AIDS is also a factor in adhering to a very demanding drug regimen without disclosing positive status in social settings (Rao et al., 2007; Ware et al., 2006). However, adherence is so important because antiretroviral therapy needs to be taken lifelong and lapses can lead to the rapid development of drug resistance, which can make future treatment much more difficult (for a discussion of adherence in diabetes care see Chapter 6). For these reasons it is hoped that pharmaceutical developments should make single dose combination therapy a reality in the near future. The toxicity of antiretrovirals relates to a number of disfiguring, debilitating and potentially fatal side effects which have been reduced as new regimens have been developed, but living with HIV is still not easy. The benefits of HAART still outweigh the disadvantages, but these challenges mean that therapy is less aggressive and initiated only when the immune system is weakened, that is the CD_4 count (a measure used to assess immune status) falls to around 200 cells/mm^3 (Gazzard and Jones, 2006). The development of antiretrovirals has also had a major impact on HIV prevention as they can be used to help prevent mother to child transmission and as a form of 'emergency' prophylaxis after exposure (within 72 hours). However, the latter is still largely reserved for health practitioners following accidental exposure rather than people who may have been put at risk through sharing injecting equipment or engaging in unprotected sex (Park, 2006).

There are some physical symptoms associated with initial HIV infection, such as flu-like symptoms and diarrhoea. However, unless the HIV remains untreated and the infection progresses so that the individual can be said to have developed AIDS, it is not really the HIV infection itself which causes the severe physical difficulties, but the treatment. There are possible serious acute side effects, and a range of short term side effects which could potentially have an initial impact on adherence (Rao et al., 2007). However, it is the long term side effects of antiretrovirals which mean that PLWHA might have to cope with chronic pain (peripheral neuropathy), changes to their physical appearance (lypodystrophy, lypoatrophy, dermatitis), endocrinological problems (high blood lipids, liver problems, diabetes, insulin resistance), as well as the complex drug regimen and the possible interactions with different foods. Although current treatment regimes are thankfully less likely to make the patient suffer the more visible side effects of HAART, the loss of subcutaneous fat which makes the face, buttocks and upper arms appear wasted (lypoatrophy) combined with fat accumulation in the abdomen, between the shoulder blades and (in women) in the breasts (lypodystrophy) can be highly distressing and seriously effect body image. Initially it was felt that PLWHA would be willing to live with the side effects and the restrictions on lifestyle that taking antiretroviral drugs entailed because it gave them a longer life, but this is not always so (Gazzard and Jones, 2006).

HIV/AIDS care in the United Kingdom

The first case of AIDS in the United Kingdom was diagnosed in 1982, and since then there have been 17,414 HIV-related deaths to the end of 2006 (HPA and HPS, 2007). The UK Health Protection Agency estimated that at the end of 2005, there are 63,500 adults (aged 15–59 years) living with HIV/AIDS in the United Kingdom, of whom 32 per cent are undiagnosed (HPA, 2006). This equates to an adult prevalence rate of approximately 0.2 per cent. There has been a recent rapid increase in the number of people being diagnosed with HIV and accessing HIV services, with around 7,000 new cases per year. There has also been a dramatic decline in the number of AIDS diagnoses since the introduction of HAART. Since 1982, 1,765 children (aged under 16 years) have also tested positive for HIV (HPA, 2006).

As is true elsewhere in northern Europe, Men Who Have Sex with Men (MSM) have been the group most affected by HIV in the United Kingdom thus far, and they are still the group at the highest risk of acquiring HIV within the United Kingdom. However, infections acquired through heterosexual intercourse have driven the rapid increase in the number of HIV diagnoses since 1997. Most of these infections were acquired overseas, and occurred among black African-born people living in the United Kingdom. In the mid-1980s there was an explosive outbreak of HIV among Injecting Drug Users (IDU), but following concerted harm reduction efforts to reduce the sharing of injecting equipment, HIV transmission among IDUs has been relatively low in the United Kingdom, especially compared with injecting drug related transmission in southern and eastern Europe. However, recent increases in hepatitis B transmission rates among IDUs would indicate that riskier injecting practices have been increasing again. More than 1,200 haemophiliacs contracted HIV through blood products before the introduction of viricidal heat treatment, and five health care workers have acquired HIV in the United Kingdom through work-related needle-stick injuries (Imrie et al., 2006).

Initially, PLWHA were treated in stand alone services and the cases were managed by specialists. Stand alone services were necessary because of the stigma and discrimination that surrounded the HIV epidemic, however, the escalation in the number of individuals seen for HIV care, together with increases in complex patient management, has put pressure on existing HIV services (HPA, 2006). The nature of the epidemic situation in the United Kingdom means that most of the people accessing HIV-related services are MSM, and the origins of these services are in 'gay friendly' sexual health clinics (Imrie et al., 2006). However, the shifting balance in the groups most affected by HIV means that services need to be appropriate for addressing the needs of people from an even wider range of different social and cultural backgrounds. Virtually all care for diagnosed PLWHA is provided by the National Health Service (NHS) through STI clinics in local hospitals, and the HIV/AIDS epidemic has brought an increase in the number of clinics, staff and resources to sexual health services in the United Kingdom, which had historically been under-resourced (Imrie et al., 2006). However, this pattern of service provision is not appropriate for children living with HIV/AIDS, where a family centered approach is needed until the young person can make the transition to adult services. Standards of care for children and young PLWHA have only recently been developed in the United Kingdom (Lyall, 2003).

The use of antiretrovirals in the treatment of HIV/AIDS in the United Kingdom began in 1988 with Zidovudine (AZT) monotherapy, which was superseded by dual therapy in the early 1990s and HAART (triple therapy) by 1996. However, antiretroviral drugs are expensive and the cost of managing a person with HIV/AIDS ranges from £10–20,000 per year and current estimates are that service providers are underfunded by approximately £3–5,000 per PLWHA per year (Imrie et al., 2006). Through the NHS, those in need, if eligible, have access to HIV treatment and care, and special provisions mean that they do not have to pay prescription charges for medications. However, eligibility is a key issue in the care for PLWHA as 'overseas visitors' (i.e., those who have not applied to remain in the United Kingdom or who are on short-stay visas) are not eligible for HIV treatment beyond testing and counselling or emergency treatment (Imrie et al., 2006). This policy is designed to discourage economic health migrants, but it throws up a whole range of issues related to definitions of essential care, prevention of long term health costs and the public health implications of PLWHA remaining outside the health system. Concerns about eligibility can also discourage people from coming forward for testing (see Erwin et al., 2002). This policy can also result in an unacceptable disruption in HIV care and treatment, especially for pregnant women in preventing vertical (mother to child) transmission.

Defining 'AIDS'

Advances in antiretroviral treatment have transformed the nature of living with HIV and they have also challenged the view of AIDS as the final stage of HIV infection. AIDS is the term used to cover a constellation of opportunistic infections and sarcomas which are associated with the deficiencies in cellular immunity caused by HIV infection. Because these particular cancers are viral in origin and relatively unusual, they are considered AIDS-defining illnesses in HIV positive people (Gazzard and Jones, 2006). HAART has helped immunodeficient individuals to boost their CD_4 count back above the boundary level used as one marker of 'full-blown' AIDS. From when the HIV antibody test became available in 1984, a small group of HIV positive people who did not develop AIDS was identified, so AIDS has never been the inevitable consequence of HIV infection, but with the advent of HAART, the distinguishing line between 'HIV positive' and 'AIDS' has been blurred beyond recognition. It is possible for a severely immuno-compromized patient to present with 'AIDS' having never received treatment for HIV infection but, with treatment, to progress from having AIDS to being HIV positive.

From a biomedical perspective, HAART is presented as a means of delaying the normal progression from HIV infection to 'full-blown' AIDS indefinitely (where patients are able to comply with the drugs regimen). However, from a sociological perspective, this final, fatal stage of normal disease progression is a construct, a way of presenting a new phenomenon as a known and predictable disease with fixed stages (Sontag, 1991). While this may have sound clinical value, it also reinforces common perceptions of what has become a long term condition as an inevitably fatal illness. HIV/AIDS is thus presented as a 'death sentence', and this association has implications for testing, treatment and care as it makes the disease more frightening to society and those carrying the disease are therefore more stigmatized. Stigma and fear of having a terminal illness can discourage people from coming forward for testing out of fatalism ('what's the point if HIV is incurable and AIDS is inevitable?') or to avoid future discrimination by confirming

HIV positive status. Even if HIV positive status has been confirmed, if attending dedicated services or the side effects are too visible, stigma will also deter people from treatment or cause problems with adherence (Rao et al., 2007; Ware et al., 2006). The roots of such stigma run deep and have been the subject of much sociological inquiry in the HIV/AIDS field.

Stigmatizing HIV/AIDS

As Goffman (1963) has argued, stigma is essentially a special kind of relationship between attribute and stereotype; a meaning imposed on an attribute via negative images, stereotypes and attitudes that potentially discredits a person (also see Chapter 1). The discredited are those whose stigma has been made visible and who have to manage the stress of this situation; the discreditable are those whose stigma remains concealed and they have to manage information and negotiate the issue of disclosure (Goffman, 1963). In this way, the stigma of HIV/AIDS is a product of the negative associations the virus has, such as a 'plague', a 'death sentence', a 'tragedy'; images which are reflected and reinforced through discourse – the forms of language used to describe something – and, by association, the people who have it (Lupton, 1994, 1999). The stigma of having HIV/AIDS thus works on two levels: externally through real discrimination in society, and internally through a sense of 'shame' at being imperfect and fear of discrimination. This fear of discrimination and 'shame' make this invisible stigmatized disease a secret which needs to be managed and concealed in order to retain a 'normal' identity.

HIV/AIDS has been imbued with apocalyptic and extremely negative characteristics that other communicable diseases with a similar prognosis if left untreated have not. HIV/AIDS is perceived as an 'especially dread disease' (Sontag, 1991). AIDS emerged at a time when apocalyptic visions of the future connected with environmental degradation and other factors were being promoted, and AIDS as a new, incurable disease was easy to frame as a 'plague' with all the biblical and moral connotations which come with it (Nettleton, 2006). AIDS first began to get noticed in human populations only in 1981, and it was first identified as a disease which affected one particular group – gay men living in San Francisco. For this reason, AIDS was first identified as Gay Related Immune Deficiency (GRID), although this was revised when it became known that the disease, while predominantly affecting one social group, was not caused by a particular lifestyle, but by a specific virus. HIV is a blood born virus which can be sexually transmitted, and the groups most seriously affected in the early days of the HIV/AIDS epidemic in the United States and Europe were MSM, IDUs, commercial sex workers and recipients of unscreened blood products. The especially negative image and consequent stigma of HIV/AIDS is related to a number of factors, but particularly its nature as a potentially sexually transmitted infection, with the associated notions of contamination and dirt and the military metaphors which have so strongly shaped the way in which HIV/AIDS has been explained.

The 'War on AIDS'

The use of military metaphor in describing novel incurable infections strikes a deep chord in society as it is a feature not just of science fiction and popular cultural visions of apocalyptic futures, but it is also central to the biological imagination (also see Chapter 10). As Waldby (1996, p. 1) has highlighted: '[E]pidemics are crisis points in the Darwinian evolutionary struggle between the microscopic, inhuman world of bacteria and viruses, and human populations. The microscopic world is on a mission to colonise the human, to render the human body an extension of the bacterial and viral interests.' Declarations of epidemic are thus declarations of war (Waldby, 1996), and the emergence of HIV/AIDS as a new epidemic in the human population meant that military metaphor was a general feature of all discourse on the subject. HIV is presented as an invisible enemy force, which invades the body, where it silently reproduces until it is strong enough to attack our defense systems from the inside (Sontag, 1991).

The invisibility of the virus (even now, the 'HIV test', is actually an antibody test, not a test for the virus itself) and the fact that most carriers exhibit no symptoms, heighten the danger. Those who secretly, and unknowingly, carry the virus are therefore to be feared as the vulnerable margin through which the disease can be contracted. The extension of military metaphor to public health campaigns was therefore not helpful. Although a 'War on AIDS' may reasonably be presented as a war on the virus, by extension it is also a war on PLWHA and even those identity categories which are associated with the virus, the 'future infected'; declarations of war allow the deployment of legitimate violence (Waldby, 1996). While many people living with long term conditions internalize military metaphor in conceptualizing their own struggle to overcome a disease or its symptoms; the use of military metaphor in public health campaigning helps to build the stigma of HIV infection and so the stigmatization of those living with HIV/AIDS.

HIV/AIDS and contamination

Once the primary transmission routes for HIV became known, it was possible to develop interventions to help prevent the disease, but this threw up major challenges for coy governments. Although Sexually Transmitted Infections (STIs) have long been the subject of public health campaigning, historically this has been conducted from a position of 'hygiene'. Although the approach is sound from a medical perspective – promoting barrier methods as a means of preventing physical contact with potentially contaminated people – it also reinforced the notion that only 'dirty' people get STIs, which is why 'clean' people need to protect themselves by not sitting on toilet seats in public lavatories, and avoiding casual contact with 'risk groups' (Sontag, 1991). Consequently, while HIV/AIDS awareness materials have consistently been clear that the virus has very specific transmission routes (predominantly anal or vaginal intercourse, transfusion of unscreened blood products, use of unsterile injecting equipment, mother to child), the stigma is such that casual contact with PLWHA is feared.

Gay men, IDUs and commercial sex workers already occupy a marginal position; they are generally stigmatized and often criminalized groups in the societies where they live. Consequently, HIV/AIDS as a disease which initially affected these groups in particular, has been framed in moral terms – as divine retribution for a sinful life in the form of a 'plague' with death sentence. HIV/AIDS is thus linked with notions of dirt and morality, as a disease which affects people who transgress notional boundaries between what is acceptable and 'clean' and what is stigmatized and 'dirty'. However, once the virus itself is framed by society as 'dirty', being HIV positive becomes the stigmatizing issue rather than the circumstances under which it is contracted (Sontag, 1991). 'Guilt' and 'innocence' instead focuses on the extent to which the individual with HIV/AIDS poses a risk to others in society, that is provided they have 'changed their ways' and turned their back on their previous sinful life (Lupton, 1999).

Lupton's (1994, 1999) work analyzing media representations of HIV/AIDS shows that media and popular discourses tend to frame PLWHA as either 'innocent victims' (e.g., haemophiliacs infected through contaminated blood products or babies born with the virus) or 'immoral' (e.g., drug users, sex workers, promiscuous heterosexuals or MSM). This innocent/ guilty divide is reinforced by the public health focus on health states which can be ameliorated by the right lifestyle choices, because it focuses on the individual's role in maintaining health (Lupton, 1999). However, all HIV positive individuals face prejudice in all aspects of their lives as carriers of an especially dread disease; where minority status is added into the mix, the prejudice is multiplied. Similarly, members of any 'high risk' group also become stigmatized as potential carriers of a dread disease. For example, although haemophiliac children would be granted innocent victimhood, once children were identified as haemophiliac they were often excluded from school irrespective of whether they were HIV positive, usually under pressure from other parents. To some extent, an HIV positive diagnosis still carries strong implications as to lifestyle, sexual preference, ethnicity and class by association with the virus, despite campaigners and public health officials arguing against such stereotyping (Park, 2006). Therefore, the disclosure of one stigmatized identity (e.g., homosexuality) infers the risk of disclosing the other, and vice versa.

In the early days of the HIV epidemic, and periodically since then, there have been calls for PLWHA to be isolated in order to protect society. This fits with the early images of HIV as a 'plague' visited upon those who had sinned, but also with notions of 'dirt', where PLWHA need to be isolated from society to avoid contamination. It links the disease into the fear of contagion and images of the leper – where the people unlucky enough to contract the disease also bore the burden of protecting society. From the very early days of the HIV epidemic, newspapers have consistently reinforced this image. However, from a public health perspective it has not made epidemiological sense, nor would it fit with European social-democratic values, to place the entire burden of HIV control on HIV positive people (Park, 2006). For this reason, the emphasis in Europe has been placed on the notion of shared responsibility between the infected and uninfected for protection. However, the burden of negotiating disclosure, non-disclosure and protection is one of the greatest challenges for PLWHA, in what is an already difficult situation (Rhodes and Cusick, 2000).

Living with HIV/AIDS

Biographical disruption

Until the advent of HAART, there was no reliable 'future' for PLWHA, and, at least for those who can access it, treatment has given PLWHA a new chance to look to the future and not just live for the moment, a chance to refine the narrative reconstructions of themselves, their condition, and their lives (Ezzy, 1998). Although there are no clear and predictable phases in the progression of HIV/AIDS, HAART can give PLWHA a sense of certainty which a positive diagnosis can undermine. It is the positive diagnosis rather than a change in abilities or sudden ill health for PLWHA which appears to have the greatest, what Bury (1982) has described as, 'biographical disruption' to their everyday world (also see Chapters 1 and 5). The way in which HIV/AIDS is perceived in society means that a positive test for HIV antibodies changes more than just a person's HIV status, they are still the same individual and they still inhabit the same body and often have the same physical abilities, but their social situation has changed, and often, so too has their relationship with their body – they have experienced biographical disruption. A positive HIV diagnosis thus becomes a part of someone's identity – potentially in how they see themselves, but predominantly in how they are viewed by others.

The experience of living with HIV/AIDS, being tested for HIV/AIDS and coping with the side effects of HAART are highly investigated areas of sociological enquiry. How the new positive status becomes a part of someone's identity depends greatly on how the person came to be infected and any pre-existing group identities they had, because people from different groups experience a positive HIV diagnosis very differently. For example, a white middle-class gay man will have different reference points, experiences and social networks to draw on than a black African refugee woman or a young person with haemophilia.

In their work on HIV positive women from Africa living in London, Anderson and Doyal (2004) found that although this group of women was far from homogenous, they had many common experiences of living with HIV including a strong need to maintain the secret of their diagnosis from fear of the stigma they may face in their communities (see also Erwin et al., 2002). However, despite HIV positive status being a secret part of their identities, many still felt that their positive diagnosis made them feel like a different person. Their problems in living with HIV were also intricately linked into the other problems they were facing in their lives as migrants. This resonates with findings from interviews with women living with HIV/AIDS in the United States; Ciambrone (2001) found that while a positive HIV diagnosis had been integrated into these women's biographies, it was just one of many disruptive life events. The women in Ciambrone's study deemed drug use, homelessness, abusive relationships and being separated from their children to be more destructive than HIV/AIDS. With hindsight, despite the lasting impact of HIV/AIDS on their future plans and goals, becoming HIV positive was not the most devastating event in these women's lives (Ciambrone, 2001).

In their work on gay men and haemophiliacs living with HIV in Paris, Carricaburu and Pierret (1995) found that all their respondents had to rework their sense of identity, through 'biographical reinforcement', that is, their identity prior to HIV infection became their preferred basis for their new identities. While asymptomatic, their HIV status was not a 'positive illness identity'. Instead, their haemophilia or homosexuality were recontextualized in the light of a positive diagnosis. Fearing the stigma of AIDS, the men with haemophilia even hid their pre-existing condition, something they would not have done before they tested positive; while the gay men tended to assert the normalcy of their homosexuality (Carricaburu and Pierret, 1995).

The epidemiological profile of HIV/AIDS in the United Kingdom shows that PLWHA are not a homogenous group. Given that HIV positive status is not generally a 'positive illness identity' and is just one of many health and social needs, it is important to ensure that care is not driven by those needs which present the greatest public health priority. Being HIV positive may not constitute a 'master status' which characterizes all aspects of PLWHA lives (Ciambrone, 2001) (also see Chapter 11 for a discussion of the concept of master status). The different ways in which living with HIV/AIDS is integrated into the biographies of PLWHA demonstrates the importance of ensuring that services and care aim to support the whole person with all the difficulties they face and not just as a case of HIV/AIDS.

Stigma and disclosure

Although advocacy groups have worked hard to reduce the stigma of living with HIV, and treatment regimes have massively improved both the quality of life and life expectancy of PLWHA, it would be wrong to imply that PLWHA lead 'normal' lives (Park, 2006). HIV remains a significant social issue for those affected. HIV discrimination is a feature of society at both an operational and structural level and managing the secret of a positive HIV status is a core concern. The issue of disclosure is one which is difficult to negotiate, because it is also linked in to notions of identity and resistance. The change a positive diagnosis for HIV, as with other long term conditions, has on an individual's self and identity is more substantial and permanent than it is for acute illness, but this may not be acknowledged or recognized at first, particularly as the condition is 'invisible' (Kelly and Field, 1996). Whereas other invisible long term conditions such as diabetes may be managed privately and successfully without any need for disclosure outside healthcare settings; HIV, as a communicable disease, makes disclosure a moral issue when sharing drugs or expressing sexuality.

In her work on women living with HIV in the United States, Ciambrone (2001) described the impact it had on her respondents as a 'sexual death'; these women's identity as desirable, sexual beings was threatened or even destroyed. In their work on HIV positive women from Africa living in London, Anderson and Doyal (2004) found that some of the women did not share their positive diagnosis with their sexual partner in order to protect themselves from verbal/physical abuse or from losing them (Anderson and Doyal, 2004). In their work on gay men and haemophiliacs living with HIV in Paris, Carricaburu and Pierret (1995) found that regardless of how they had become infected, all interviewees decided to tell no-one of their status except a few people to whom they were very close because the stigma of HIV was so great. The stigma of HIV contributes to many difficulties in coping with treatment regimens, but it can also create much greater difficulties in negotiating safer sexual practices and condom use (Vanable et al., 2006). The legacy of HIV/AIDS being perceived as something which generally affects 'immoral' people and as a 'death sentence' has significant repercussions for PLWHA and their decision to disclose their HIV positive status, to whom, when and how.

Criminalization of 'reckless' transmission in the United Kingdom

Disclosure is an increasingly important issue for PLWHA, particularly in the United Kingdom, because the accessibility of HAART has shifted the nature of living with HIV from a 'death sentence' to a 'long term condition' requiring medication. This has coincided with an epidemiological shift which has seen growing rates of heterosexual transmission relative to homosexual transmission in the United Kingdom. This epidemiological shift has been accompanied by the criminalization of 'reckless' HIV transmission in the United Kingdom through the successful prosecution of individuals living with HIV/AIDS who did not disclose their status to sexual partners who went on to test positive for HIV antibodies. While disclosing known HIV positive status to sexual partners may be the most ethically defensible practice, 'what is ethically warranted is not necessarily what the law mandates or ought to mandate' (Wealt and Azad, 2005, p. 9). This legal development actually serves to reinforce the stigma of HIV/AIDS and minority groups, particularly through media reporting, and undermines the fundamental sexual health message that HIV prevention should be based on shared responsibility in the face of sexual risk (Park, 2006).

In Scotland, England and Wales, since the legalist approach to HIV was established in 2001, there have been nine successful prosecutions: two women and seven men, one of whom was gay. The two women and six of the men were prosecuted for transmitting HIV to their heterosexual partners; three of these men were of black African origin. In Scotland the prosecution was for 'reckless injury' while in England and Wales people were charged with 'recklessly inflicting grievous bodily harm' due to transmission of HIV under section 20 of the Offences Against the Person Act 1861. Despite media reports, none of the convictions have been for intentional harm; such a conviction would involve a much heavier burden of proof. These prosecutions mean that in sexual relations between consenting adults, the responsibility is not on the uninfected individual for protecting their own health, nor is it shared between two sexual partners; in law the person living with HIV is entirely responsible. Moreover, as one of the people convicted had never had an HIV antibody test, being a member of a 'risk group', such as black African, is thus sufficient for prosecution, as the person could reasonably have expected to be HIV positive. The potential for the legalist model to feed discrimination is clear. In the broader policy context, there is a worrying trend towards coercive responses to HIV through criminalization, but also through debates around compulsory testing following alleged criminal incidents or of new migrants (Wealt and Azad, 2005).

The image of the 'AIDS carrier' as a duplicitous individual who carelessly or maliciously spreads HIV to others is not new to the media. The image conforms to elements of 'epidemic psychology' or the feelings of fear, suspicion, panic and the need to take strong action against the scapegoats, which emerges when an epidemic emerges and appears to threaten society (Lupton, 1999). Those charged with reckless transmission have been charged because they have reacted inappropriately to their positive diagnosis – instead of 'learning their lesson' in the face of their 'divine retribution for a dissolute lifestyle', reforming their life and facing their condition bravely, they carried on as before. 'These individuals' inability or lack of willingness to contain their bodies was represented as dangerous and contaminating, and they were therefore subject to moral censure.' (Lupton, 1999, p. 51) However, it is not clear that such legislation is in the interests of the public health – there is no indication that criminalization prevents the transmission of HIV/AIDS either through fear of punishment or isolation. However, the further stigmatization of PLWHA is certainly unhelpful for prevention efforts (Galletly and Pinkerton, 2006; Wealt and Azad, 2005).

Conclusion

To a certain extent, developments in treatment options for PLWHA might help to reduce the stigma of HIV, but improved knowledge is known to have the greatest impact on stigmatization. For example, one study, which investigated the process of stigmatization in health care settings, showed that the fear of contagion and subsequent negative reaction to PLWHA by health care workers declined as health professionals became more familiar with treating them (Green and Platt, 1997). This shows how health professionals can reinforce or challenge prevailing stigma in society, but their impact on HIV care and prevention can be even more profound through a recognition of the diversity within this 'illness group'. The impact of HIV on people's lives is relative to the other negative events they have survived or endured. Not everyone who is diagnosed as HIV positive has the same level of support and not everyone has the same needs – HIV might not have 'master status' in their identity or conceptualization of their health. Understanding the fuller complexity of different people's needs in relation to their HIV positive status is essential for developing effective treatment protocols – particularly in view of the complex nature of HAART. It is also important for developing suitable prevention efforts and ensuring that the legislative and policy framework is appropriate for promoting the public health and not just for reinforcing the stigma of HIV/AIDS.

Within health services, nurses are most often the first point of contact for PLWHA and they are the staff members who bear the greatest responsibility for the on-going treatment and care in the community for those living with this long term condition. Comprehensive nursing care for PLWHA incorporates clinical management of the condition, direct patient care, education, prevention, counselling, palliative care and social support for adults, families and children. Nurses are thus uniquely well placed to ensure that greater understanding of the complexity of people's needs is integrated into the continuum of care for PLWHA and to help challenge the stigma such individuals face.

References

Anderson J., and L. Doyal, 'Women from Africa living with HIV in London: a descriptive study', *AIDS Care*, 16: 1 (2004) 95–105.

Bury M., 'Chronic illness as biographical disruption', *Sociology of Health and Illness*, 4: 2 (1982) 451–468.

Carricaburu D., and J. Pierret, 'From biographical disruption to biographical reinforcement: The case of HIV positive men', *Sociology of Health and Illness*, 17: 1 (1995) 65–88.

Ciambrone D., 'Illness and other assaults on self: the relative impact of HIV/AIDS on women's lives', *Sociology of Health and Illness*, 23: 4 (2001) 517–540.

Erwin J., M. Morgan, N. Britten, K. Gray and B. Peters, 'Pathways to HIV testing and care by black African and white patients in London', *Sexually Transmitted Infections*, 78 (2002) 37–39.

Ezzy D., 'Lived experience and interpretation in narrative theory: Experiences of living with HIV/AIDS', *Qualitative Sociology*, 21: 2 (1998) 169–179.

Fleet J., and B. N'Daw, 'Trade, intellectual property and access to affordable HIV medications', in E.J. Beck et al. (eds), *The HIV Pandemic: Local and Global Implications* (New York: Oxford University Press, 2006).

Galletly C.L., and S.D. Pinkerton, 'Conflicting messages: how criminal HIV disclosure laws undermine public health efforts to control the spread of HIV', *AIDS and Behavior*, 10: 5 (2006) 451–461.

Gazzard B.G., and R.S. Jones, 'From death to life: two decades of progress in HIV therapy', in S. Matic, J.V. Lazarus and M.C. Donoghoe (eds), *HIV/AIDS in Europe: Moving from Death Sentence to Chronic Disease Management* (Copenhagen: WHO Regional Office for Europe, 2006).

Goffman E., *Stigma: Notes on the Management of Spoiled Identity* (Harmondsworth: Penguin Books, 1963).

Green G., and S. Platt, 'Fear and loathing in health care settings reported by people with HIV', *Sociology of Health and Illness*, 19: 1 (1997) 70–92.

Health Protection Agency [HPA], The UK Collaborative Group for HIV and STI Surveillance, *A Complex Picture. HIV and other Sexually Transmitted Infections in the United Kingdom: 2006* (London: Health Protection Agency, Centre for Infections: November 2006).

Health Protection Agency [HPA] Centre for Infections and Health Protection Scotland [HPS], Unpublished Quarterly Surveillance Tables No. 75, 07/2 (London: Health Protection Agency, Centre for Infections, July 2007) http://www.hpa.org.uk/infections/topics_az/hiv_and_sti/hiv/epidemiology/files/Quarterlies%202007/2007_Q2_(Jun)_HIV_Quarterlies.pdf (last accessed 5 October 2007).

Imrie J., S. Dougan, K. Gray, M.W. Adler, A.M. Johnson, B.G. Evans and B.S. Peters, 'The United Kingdom', in E.J. Beck et al. (eds), *The HIV Pandemic: Local and Global Implications* (New York: Oxford University Press, 2006).

Kelly M.P., and D. Field, 'Medical sociology, chronic illness and the body', *Sociology of Health and Illness*, 18: 2 (1996) 241–257.

Lange J.M.A., 'Antiretroviral treatment and care of HIV', in E.J. Beck et al. (eds), *The HIV Pandemic: Local and Global Implications* (New York: Oxford University Press, 2006).

Lupton D., *Moral Threats and Dangerous Desires: AIDS in the New Media* (London: Taylor and Francis, 1994).

Lupton D., 'Archetypes of infection: people with HIV/AIDS in the Australian press in the mid 1990s', *Sociology of Health and Illness*, 21: 1 (1999) 37–53.

Lyall H., *Growing Up, Gaining Independence – Principles for Transition of HIV Care* (London: Children's HIV Association of UK and Ireland (CHIVA), 2003) *http://www.chiva.org.uk/protocols/ adolescence.html* (last accessed 18 April 2007).

Nettleton S., *The Sociology of Health and Illness*, 2nd edn (Cambridge: Polity Press, 2006).

C. Park, 'Empowering people living with HIV in Europe: manifesto, mantra or mirage?', in S. Matic, J.V. Lazarus and M.C. Donoghoe (eds), *HIV/AIDS in Europe: Moving from Death Sentence to Chronic Disease Management* (Copenhagen: WHO Regional Office for Europe, 2006).

Rao D., T.C. Kekwaletswe, S. Hosek, J. Martinez and F. Rodriguez, 'Stigma and social barriers to medication adherence with urban youth living with HIV', *AIDS Care*, 19: 1 (2007) 28–33.

Rhodes T., and L. Cusick 'Love and intimacy in relationship risk management: HIV positive people and their sexual partners', *Sociology of Health and Illness*, 22: 1 (2000) 1–26.

Sontag S., *Illness as Metaphor and AIDS and Its Metaphors* (London: Penguin Books, 1991).

Vanable P.A., M.P. Carey, D.C. Blair, R.A. Littlewood, 'Impact of HIV-related stigma on health related behaviors and psychological adjustment among HIV-positive men and women', *AIDS and Behavior*, 10: 5 (2006) 473–482.

Waldby C., *AIDS and the Body Politic: Biomedicine and Sexual Difference* (London and New York: Routledge, 1996).

Ware N.C., M.A. Wyatt and T. Tungenberg, 'Social relationships, stigma and adherence to antiretroviral therapy for HIV/AIDS', *AIDS Care*, 18: 8 (2006) 904–910.

Wealt M., and Y. Azad, 'The criminalization of HIV transmission in England and Wales: questions of law and policy', *HIV/AIDS Policy & Law Review*, 10: 2 (2005) 1–12.

World Health Organization [WHO], UNAIDS and UNICEF, *Towards Universal Access: Scaling up Priority HIV/AIDS Interventions in the Health Sector: Progress Report* (Geneva: WHO, April 2007).

9 Witness and duty: answering the call to speak for dementia sufferers in advanced illness

Pauline Savy

Introduction

Dementing illness in old age brings profound challenges for sufferers[1] and for those who care for them. Relentless deterioration of mental and physical capacities makes the illness a human tragedy in the fullest sense: over time, everything that constitutes the social existence of sufferers crumbles. Nearing the end of their illness, sufferers may become incoherent or mute. They may live on in a vegetative state seemingly unaware of the significance of people and things around them. Terms such as 'silhouettes' or 'shells', (Anderson, 1986; Yingling, 1985) have been poetically used to describe this seemingly empty existence. Similarly used, the stark metaphor 'living death' reflects perceptions that sufferers are biologically alive but mentally and socially dead, or, more ambiguously, they are neither alive nor dead.

For family members and friends, this state is a painful mystery for little may be left of the person they once knew. What makes this loss particularly heartbreaking is that selfhood in dementia can be at once elusive and apparent. On the one hand, dementia strips away identifying personal characteristics, but, on the other hand, it may lay bare, or even accentuate, enduring and endearing traits and habits that speak of the person, past and present. Occasional familiar gestures, facial expressions and turns of phrase may remind others of who the person once was. Or, still might be.

Equally for nurses, the problem of unraveling selfhood is a mysterious matter. Patients are often admitted to care when their family and friends consider them to no longer be the person they once knew. At the same time, contemporary care ethics charge nurses with getting to know patients and confirming their selfhood. That is, dementia care is caught up in discourses or 'stories' of selfhood. I make the point in this chapter that while the nursing 'voice' as it speaks for patients is undoubtedly, ethically enhanced by these discourses, there remains space for a parallel story that tells of the *deep plight* (Bruner, 2002) of severely demented patients. And that space awaits the voices of nurses, who in their special roles of *witness* and *duty* (Frank, 1995) are subjectively entangled in that story.

In this chapter, I elaborate the problem of selfhood for dementia sufferers, particularly for individuals whose advanced illness prevents speaking coherently for themselves. I begin by setting out the discourses of selfhood in dementia that surround and shape the obligations of contemporary professional caregiving. I then go on to locate the problems of sufferers' selfhood in advanced dementia and nursing care within the concept of *existential labour* (Gubrium, 1986). This concept goes to the heart of nurses' ambiguous relationships with, and duty towards, such patients. Significantly, it provides language to describe the plight of sufferers, the phenomenal terrain of dementia care, and the possibilities for and limits to discursively producing sufferers' selfhood.

Finally, I propose that nurses are well placed within roles of *duty* and *witness* (Frank, 1995) to produce accounts of dementing illness, particularly narratives that speak of the subjective worlds of illness and care in advanced dementia. Thus, they may contribute much-needed 'bottom-up' accounts that represent more 'near-ly' these worlds. This work will necessarily expand narrative methodologies for writing about individuals who are unable to speak for themselves, and who exist liminally between culturally-defined categories of life and death.

Discourses of dementia: self lost and discoverable

Over the last four decades, the literature on dementia has burgeoned. The theoretical and practical matters raised in this literature revolve around the problem of who the person is, or can be, as the illness advances. Two broad understandings of this problem can be elicited. On one hand, the dominant, bio-medical view of dementia portrays sufferers as 'lost' to disease. On the other hand, a psychosocial view suggests that selfhood or personhood is not necessarily lost, that it can be discovered and preserved right through to the late stages of the illness. Both conclusions can be found across social science analyses.

For my purposes, I sort the literature into biomedical, psychosocial, and social science categories. However, the distinctions are not always clear-cut as overlaps exist across illness descriptions, and across authors' intentions and conclusions. Some sociological analyses, for example, mirror concerns in the psychosocial literature and advocate care techniques that act towards selfhood. I do not single out the nursing literature for discussion here although this constitutes a vast and valuable body of work that straddles both biomedical and psychosocial orientations in its concern with therapeutic and dignifying care approaches.

The loss of self in the biomedical literature

The biomedical literature primarily depicts dementing illness as a disease of the brain, a bleak and depersonalizing, self-stripping disorder wrought by devastating and irreversible pathology. Dementia is often referred to as a syndrome, or complex of symptoms, that results from global cerebral destruction such as that associated with Alzheimer's, Parkinson's and cerebrovascular diseases. The impairments are usually summarized as increasing decline in cognitive, emotional and perceptual-motor abilities that are integral to the functions of memory, abstract thinking, judgment, and other complex capabilities such as speech and language, the ability to carry out complex physical tasks, and recognition of objects and people (Mace, 1987). Additionally, symptoms may include mental and behavioural disorders such as confusion, delusional thought, depression and impulsive emotional outbursts.

Impairments are described as insidious at first and easily mistaken as senile changes. Over time they become more obvious and more disabling as mental alertness wanes and periods of confusion and disorientation diminish capacity to manage the personal and social matters of daily life. Degenerative changes accumulate for some ten or more years until finally sufferers become mute, inattentive, immobile and completely dependent upon others (Maas et al., 1994). Within the biomedical model, the course of dementia is often organized into stages that imply typical progression, predictability and manageability. Illness progression is commonly understood through terms such as 'early' and 'advanced' that represent phases of deterioration of particular abilities such as memory and orientation. However, the notion of typical progression in illnesses such as Alzheimer's disease is contradicted within the biomedical model itself by the acknowledgment that disease manifestation is generally more individual than uniform (Cohen, 1991).

The disease view pervades cultural awareness through media reports that speak of dementing illness as an epidemic, a plague that takes the shine off longevity. Similarly, when personal accounts of the illness are publicized, they tend to support the disease model of declining and lost selfhood. Stories about nursing homes and dementia care settings are often mediated through sensational images of helpless, incomprehensible old folk forsaken by families and badly treated by heartless carers and tight-fisted governments. At the same time, the biomedical model of dementia contributes substantial clinical structure to nursing practice and prompts useful questions for nursing research. Clinical practice based on sound and up-to-date knowledge of the pathology that underlies and differentiates dementing illnesses is essential for the development of nursing strategies to manage specific symptoms and functional deficits. This knowledge is also necessary for researchers who want to spend time with and interview dementia sufferers. Ethical nursing practice is also served by an alternative discourse which I now set out.

Persistent selfhood in the psychosocial literature

Over the last two decades, a strong critique of the biomedical explanation of dementia has developed to reject the biomedical model's portrayal of sufferers as passive victims of relentless, de-selfing, pathology (Estes and Binney, 1989; Harding and Palfrey, 1997; Woods, 2001). A principal aim of this literature is to contextualize the illness socially and subjectively. Specifically, it aims to de-stigmatize and humanize the condition, and to re-write our means of understanding it and providing care (Downs, 1996; Lyman, 1989).

In this literature, grim pathological versions are replaced with social and psychologistic explanations of the illness in terms of aetiology and individual manifestations. One suggestion for example, is that dementing illness may ensue from a pre-morbid personality type (Kitwood, 1990). Some authors equate personality style with variance of experience and symptom intensity within and across individuals (Bender and Cheston, 1997). Behaviours such as wandering, seeking long-dead parents, and withdrawal are all explained as psychological responses rather than the direct result of cerebral pathology (Bender and Cheston, 1997; Feil, 1982; Miesen, 1992; Monsour and Robb, 1982; Shoemaker, 1987).

A pervasive idea in this literature holds that the sufferer's personhood is preservable even in advanced dementia (Kitwood and Bredin, 1992; Sabat and Harré, 1992). The social genesis of personhood is emphasized rather than its manifestation as rationality, self-awareness and individual agency. Thus, it is the task of others to fill out gestures or part-actions of sufferers so that they become meaningful social actions (Kitwood, 1993). In various ways, this task is set out in care approaches such as activity, reality orientation, reminiscence and validation therapies. In these approaches, a focus on the talk of dementia sufferers supports the idea of hidden but unique and recoverable personhood. Sufferers' remembrances are taken to be expressions of identity and analyzed as illness narratives. Listeners are directed to make sense of jumbled stories by seeking metaphoric rather than literal meanings especially when sufferers can no longer observe conventions for language use and conversation (Bohling, 1991; Cheston, 1996; Crisp, 1992; Killick and Allan, 2002; Mills, 1997; Sabat and Harré, 1992).

Critiques of the psychosocial approach, its claims and methodologies, are few. Presumably this is because its strong advocacy for person-centred care reflects broader cultural ideals concerning selfhood and consumer rights (Adams, 1996; Savy, 2004). Psychosocial arguments have opened spaces for the voices of dementia sufferers and for others to speak for them. Concepts of selfhood such as self-awareness, subjectivity, and personal experience provide language for such elaboration. These same concepts are fundamental to the social science literature to which I now turn.

The social science literature: selfhood socially realizable

From different theoretical orientations, and at different levels of enquiry, social science work generally concerns the social identity and selfhood of dementia sufferers. Studies that specifically explore the problem of sufferers' social disconnectedness and interactional ineptness frequently proceed from the theory of symbolic interactionism which establishes the self as a socially realized and individualizing entity (e.g., Fontana and Smith, 1989; Savy, 2004; Vittoria, 1999). Drawing from the early symbolic interactionism of Mead (1934) and Blumer (1969) as well as from the later contributions of Erving Goffman (1959, 1963) researchers examine the social implications of sufferers' interactions.

Goffman's dramaturgical theory of ordinary, self-negotiating interactions is a popular choice for analyzing sufferers' relations with others. From this perspective, sufferers become increasingly less able to honour conventions for ordinary interactions over the course of illness. Specifically, biographical memory fails along with the skills necessary for presenting a coherent self, for taking the role of the other, and for collaboratively constructing meaning. When they fail to meet culturally and situationally defined expectations, sufferers' identities are said to be *spoilt* through the *discrediting* or *stigmatizing* interpretations of others (Luken, 1987; Sabat and Harré, 1992). Goffman's concept of stigma is widely used across the psychosocial and the social science literature. Less acknowledged is Goffman's reference to the ameliorative work of nurses and others who manage and play down the potentially discrediting implications of sufferers' unconventional behaviours (Goffman, 1963).

Where the concept of *stigma* is used in this expanded sense it shows the restorative, socially inclusive actions of others (see for example Blum, 1991; Bogdan and Taylor, 1987; Shifflett and Blieszner, 1988).

Several analyses dwell on the ways that carers in institutional settings go about normalizing sufferers' behaviours (Fontana and Smith, 1989; Ramanathan-Abbott, 1994; Sabat and Harré, 1992; Vittoria, 1999). For example, Vittoria (1999) observed the ways that staff of a special care dementia unit discursively produced a view of sufferers' selfhood as rational by substituting words such as 'wandering' with 'busy' and 'moving' (Vittoria, 1999). Fontana and Smith (1989) observed similar normalizing strategies at the dementia day care centre they studied. From a strictly symbolic interactionist perspective, these authors conclude that dementia sufferers in this setting were token social actors whose performances consisted merely of over-learned social rules and behaviours. Acting as agents, staff assigned to them 'the last remnants of self' (Fontana and Smith, 1989, p. 45).

Similarly, in their analysis of care in an Israeli nursing home, Golander and Raz (1996) propose that work to restore selfhood may be composed of more fabrication than validation. They present examples of staff making flippant and dismissive interpretations based on biographical fragments. Such critical analyses show that attempts to salvage sufferers' selfhood, although in accord with 'filling out' approaches (Kitwood, 1993), may become awkward and ultimately subversive. They serve to emphasize rather than overcome sufferers' otherness, their social remoteness.

As a result of the psychosocial movement, empirical and other studies of sufferers themselves are now stacking up. Phenomenological, socio-linguistic, narrative and interactionist-oriented studies set out to grasp the lived, embodied experiences and the self-awareness of sufferers who are able to participate in interviews (for example Crisp, 1992, 1995; Hamilton, 1994; Harris and Sterin, 1999; Holst and Hallberg, 2003; Phinney, 1998, 2002; Phinney and Chesla, 2003; Sabat and Harré, 1992; Surr, 2006). Such studies bring a sense of order to informants' words and narratives inasmuch as their selfhood is located and described in the *language of method* followed by the researcher (Gubrium and Holstein, 1997). Sufferers, and their experiences of illness, thus become understandable through the production of a disciplined, followable story.

However, the problem of producing a coherent account of the existence, experiences and selfhood of sufferers in advanced illness who are incoherent or silent, has so far received little attention. Presumably, research at this stage has been avoided because the task to grasp and represent the lives of such disordered individuals appears difficult. In the social sciences, most theoretical and methodological means for eliciting and talking about selfhood are predicated on coherent talk and interaction. The kind of data that is likely to be elicited may comprise little more than fragmented, condensed, often wordless exchanges, images and feelings. Interpretation of this kind of material situates the researcher's subjective self at the centre of the work, a place with little formal methodological and theoretical shelter.

Thus, stories of advanced dementia, and the encompassing worlds of caregiving, remain to be explored as do the methodological means for doing so. I propose that nurses are ideally placed to attend to this research gap. In the following two sections, I explore the notions of *existential labour* (Gubrium, 1986) and *duty* and *witness* (Frank, 1995) along with the narrative concept to show how these may frame, that is, provide language and structure for the task.

Existential labour in advanced dementia

The concept of *existential labour* refers to the discursive work involved in articulating, realizing and finally, giving up on the selfhood of dementia sufferers (Gubrium, 1986). *Existential labour* is a central idea in Gubrium's analysis of how members of an Alzheimer's support group speak of the existence and selfhood of sufferers in their care (Gubrium, 1986). Following Mead's (1934) explication of socially realized selfhood, Gubrium concludes that the self, when articulated in dementia, is more fully social because of the intense and increasingly overt nature of the work that goes into its production.

Gubrium's analysis draws attention not only to the conditions and materials available to direct *existential labour*, but to the limits of its use. Materials include *articulation rules* or the rules of thumb for eliciting the minds and selfhood of sufferers (Gubrium, 1986). For example, in long term care settings the rules for talk that substantiates sufferers' selfhood can be found in prescriptive materials such as textbooks, organizational manuals, training videos, and within local sets of meanings that shape care values and practice in the setting. Where these materials charge caregivers to regard their patients as individuals whose abilities, dignities, and selfhood are preservable, they reflect the ideas of the psychosocial literature described earlier, and in turn, prevalent cultural ideologies of selfhood.

The notion of *existential labour* elaborates the problem of making something of flimsy selfhood as the illness strips away the ability to talk coherently, and leads ultimately to silence. Gubrium refers to the cessation of restorative work as 'closing off affairs with the hopelessly demented' when the demise of mind must finally be accepted, and the work of minding, or assigning self, becomes burdensome (Gubrium, 1986, p. 48). In long term care settings the 'burdens' of persisting with the work of assigning self may be socially contoured and evaluated in different terms. Sociologically, it could be said that the exaggeration and visibility of staff efforts to assign selfhood reveal sufferers' selves to be close to failure rather than to be revivable. The imminence of this failure uncovers what is at stake for the categories and practices that nursing staff construct to establish the care milieu as meaningful and purposeful. In special care units where staff understand the setting as a place for finding and restoring selfhood, sufferers will eventually be seen to be beyond the reach of such work. Relocation to a place for irredeemable cases is necessary to re-establish the taken-for-granted reality of the setting as a place where selfhood is restored (Savy, 2004; Vittoria, 1999).

In places where sufferers stay until they die, staff strategies to effect closure include task orientation to care and dismissal of sufferers' self-references and self-claims as symptoms. Such interpretations effect a degree of detachment from the profound and disturbing questions posed by the neither-dead-nor-alive existence of severely demented individuals. Still, efforts to effect closure don't cleanly resolve the ambiguities of sufferers' self-identity as they live on in a vegetative, liminal state, and in a social context.

For this discussion, the relevance of the notion of *existential labour* lies in what it says about the marginality of caregiving work in dementia, especially in advanced illness. As a meaning-making endeavour, *existential labour* takes place at the fragile, phenomenal edges of unconventional, interpersonal interactions, and of knowing. Here, nurses are likely to experience the paired nursing roles of witness and duty in terms of questions that are difficult to answer. Who are their patients? Who can they be to their patients? How can they speak for their patients and speak meaningfully about their plight?

The call to speak: witness and duty in late-stage dementing illness

> Social scientists have long given too much weight to verbalizations at the expense of visualization, to language at the expense of images.
>
> *(Bruner, 1986, p. 5)*

Edward Bruner's words encourage creativity in addressing the questions that incoherence and silence pose for care and for research. In this section, I suggest that the narrative concept can be applied to give voice to spoken and unspoken dimensions of sufferers' worlds of illness, including others' subjective, human connectedness to them. I explore conceptualizations from the work of two theorists, Frank (1995, 2001) and Hydén (1997) and exemplify their use with material selected from my ethnographic study of the experiences of dementia sufferers in three Australian long term care settings. My aim is to highlight and respond to the methodological difficulties encountered in grasping and analyzing encounters and interactions with late-stage sufferers. Eliciting and using such material inevitably raises questions about the ethics of researching severely impaired and vulnerable individuals. However, a meaningful discussion of the issues relating to consent and the philosophical and practical challenges that materialized as a result of my informants' disabilities is beyond the scope of this chapter.

The concepts of *witness* and *duty* (Frank, 1995) make a fruitful starting point to talk about the nurse-patient relationship in late-stage dementia care; they open possibilities for nurses to speak about, and for, sufferers. Witness, according to Frank, requires giving testimony to illness in the form of illness narratives. Frank sees that the ill person 'bears responsibility for telling what happened', and that immediate others have a duty to take up the call made by the narrative, that is, to act morally towards it (Frank, 1995, p. 137). For the telling, Frank's (1995) typology of illness narratives offers analytical categories that await and interpret storylines in terms of restitution, quest and chaos. *Restitution* and *quest narratives* speak of moving towards recovery or reconciliation with illness. As narratives of selfhood, they compel and inspire others. The *chaos narrative* tells of time without sequence. It turns on futility, impotence and vulnerability, and thus tells of self in disarray. These three types give structure to, and render narrative material understandable and typical in terms of the course and process of illness as they convey its meanings for the afflicted person (Hydén, 1997).

First-hand telling is problematic for dementia sufferers unable to competently account for, or give witness to their own illness experience. However, the call to give testimony can be taken up by those in the next circle of witnesses (Frank, 1995). This duty involves speaking of the illness, and for the ill individual, from the inter-human perspective of being a potentially suffering body. Speaking from this position requires a particular relationship, one 'that takes place outside of the language of survival' (Frank, 1995, p. 145). Further to this, I suggest that articulation of illness in late-stage dementia should take place outside of prevalent discourses of whole and recovering selfhood. And following Frank (2001), analytical methodologies should be used minimally and critically to show the illness experience as inherently resistant to conceptual categories. In practice, this resistance is palpable in the subjective, materials that nurses work with to know their patients. Conceptually, these can be expressed as *liminal narrativity* (Savy, 2006), or in-between materials for interpretation, as they cross and smudge the edges of knowing and not knowing, temporality and atemporality, living and dying.

Conceptual flexibility for this work can be found in Hydén's (1997) narrative categories: illness *as* narrative, narrative *about* illness and narrative *as* illness. As outlined in Chapter 1, these categories reflect the '*formal* aspects of illness narratives, namely the relationship between narrator, illness and narrative' rather than the storylines they follow (Hydén, 1997, p. 54, original emphasis). The first category locates narrator, illness and narrative in the one person and thus seems to require a speaker able to observe conventions for storytelling. However, a lateral understanding of telling allows for the ill person's body to bear witness (Frank, 1995). For example, I observed and recorded such telling in my study of incoherent and silent dementia sufferers. The following excerpt shows my approach to portraying what I saw, heard and felt in my interactions with one sufferer who could no longer speak:

> In fleeting exchanges as I held Lyla's skeletal body, her whispery breath on my neck, the hollows of her illness told me of me her nearness to collapse, the emptiness to come. Against Lyla's frailty I felt the strength of my own body and life, and my inability to help her.

Hydén's second type, narratives *about* illness, conveys knowledge and explanations of sickness, so they are often used by practitioners to construct and convey clinical knowledge (Hydén, 1997). Cases constructed thus are paradigmatic when they fit a biomedical template of disease but these accounts do not necessarily exclude practitioners' empathy. Instead, knowledge of devastating pathology may move pratcitioners subjectively towards patients' suffering. Thus, clinical narratives in dementia may tell of illness while confirming disease. Descriptions of bodily frailty, mental confusion and distress are compelling means of telling about illness. In the following tract, my analysis shows how I 'knew' Ernie whose physical and mental deterioration had made him a stranger to his family, and to himself. By referring to his bodily decline and clinical conditions, I show not only the disruptions and hardships caused by pathology, but something of the man he once was, and something of what is left to constitute his illness, and his humanity:

> Ernie's body is slackened by age and illness but he looks as if he may once have been a strong, stocky man. His freckled and roughened complexion tells of years of working outdoors in the Australian climate. One of Ernie's eyes is clouded by cataract. Indeed, he is blind. But his 'good' eye sparkles enough for both when he talks and when he laughs. And he laughs often. And I laugh with him.

Hydén's third type, narrative *as* illness, refers to conditions in which patients lack the speech, language and comprehension to tell of their experiences and to link events connected with illness. Thus narrative *as* illness is an especially useful category for framing analysis of the muddled talk and silences of dementia sufferers. The unspeakability of suffering (Frank, 2001; Hydén, 1997) and sufferers' language and speech problems do not preclude taking their jumbled words as narrative material and conveying their plight. For example, Dolly, another of my informants would more or less follow conventions for conversation but her ability to think and talk coherently fluctuated. The following analytical passage shows that sometimes there is a 'real' story in muddled talk. Importantly, the story reveals the anguish that Dolly experienced as a result of her illness:

> Over several months, Dolly's stories inferred a sorry childhood spent in an orphanage and personal tragedies of her adulthood including the loss of two children. Each telling was differently and metaphorically constructed, but in each telling, the same themes appeared. Ultimately, Dolly's daughter verified these themes as reflective of Dolly's past life. I saw them as a source of present suffering because of Dolly's inability to will away overwhelming memories and emotions. Her rogue memories seemed to fill spaces vacated by other memories – a layer of tragedy that I hadn't previously considered.

These three examples fit with Frank's suggestion that stories can be 'told around' illness and suffering (Frank, 1995). To tell around illness implies the use of materials other than the ill person's verbal account of experience. Even silent sufferers have something to tell us and articulation of the liminal world they experience can be made via other knowledge-structures such as textual representations and images that metaphorically portray the subjective and embodied experience of illness (Kirmayer, 2000). Such work depicting illness and suffering in dementia is modeled in folk poetry and anthologies (see for example Gubrium, 1988; Killick and Cordonnier, 2000).

Scholarly analyses of silence are few but they are instructive in that they modify and expand the narrative concept and methodology to capture non-literal meanings in incoherent talk and silence (examples include Booth and Booth, 1996; Lovell, 1997; Peake, 2004; Robilliard, 1997; Savy, 2004; van Dongen, 2004). These analyses are achieved through imaginative projections into illness, 'readings' of ill bodies, and styles of writing that evoke unspeakable suffering. Whilst these accounts have been assembled to meet disciplinary requirements for coherence and intellectual rigour, they remain clear examples of researchers entering and attending to potential but unrealizable narratives (Kirmayer, 2000). That is, unrealizable by following methodological conventions that aim for a satisfying sense of wholeness.

The following example describes my approach to capturing and bringing to words one sufferer's liminal illness experience. Lyla could not speak but her body was far from silent. As Lyla paced around the setting, her emaciated body bore life and death in appalling unity. In the first, ethnographically descriptive part of my analysis I inserted only three poetic entries to portray Lyla's existence in a fragmented and fragile present, as life in the breach, awaiting further fall. These sparse entries are intended to reflect the limits to knowing her in conventional ways; they show my nervous hand in the narrative. One entry describes Lyla's physical presence in the setting as at once moving towards and away from others as if to emphasize the problem of grasping and speaking about the meanings of her life:

> Round and round
> Lyla cut our circle with her own
> Through us, away and back again
> into Rhoda's hug, another circle
> to push against...

In two subsequent sections I construct denser levels of analysis, ultimately invoking Kristeva's (1982) concept of *the abject* to tell of the problem of knowing Lyla, to speak of her existence and to evoke her experience. The following two excerpts show my attempts to give substance to the *liminal narrativity* of Lyla's silence and her physical expression of illness:

> Lyla had no words of her own from which we could establish the to and fro of an ordinary relationship. Without talk I felt more like an on-looker than a participant in her life. Still, Lyla's silence held a fullness, a latency that beckoned me. Everything about Lyla, her appearance, her pacing, her resistance, I found compelling and connecting. With a paired sense of aversion and absorption I would describe Lyla as a spectre in motion between life and death, on the edge.
>
> Kristeva's (1982) concept of the abject body, horrifically out of control in serious illness, provides imagery for conveying Lyla's extreme, corpse-like appearance. The term also gives language for thinking about Lyla's self; the boundaries it once normatively constructed and policed between body and mind, rationality and emotionality, order and disorder, had broken down. In Kristevan terms, Lyla shows us the horror of dementia through the image of a body disconnected from mind.

My account cannot contain Lyla's words but it is still an illness narrative that locates her plight within an overarching, existential narrative of human frailty, loss and death; it speaks of the unspeakable. My use of Kristeva's (1982) concept of abjection marks the narrative as an academic construction. At the same time, its language allows me to keeps open the marginality and ambiguities of Lyla's experience rather than corset them in analytic categories that imply coherence and understandability.

Conclusion

In this chapter I set out to expand the existing space in the literature for speaking about illness and care in advanced dementia. Firstly, I summarized existing bodies of literature in terms of their explanations of selfhood and experience in dementing illness. The particular perspectives of the biomedical, psychosocial and social science paradigms elaborate in their own ways the complex problem of selfhood and caregiving in dementia. I then singled out the concept of *existential labour* (Gubrium, 1986) to show its value for understanding the problematic, micro-dimensions of assigning self to very impaired individuals.

To date, the literature offers little research into the subject-ive worlds of late-stage dementia sufferers. I related this gap to the methodological discomfort that arises when incoher-ent and silent individuals are regarded as informants and to the unconventional nature of the 'data' elicited in encounters with them. In response, I referred to work that attends to the unspeakable dimensions of severe illness and suffering (Booth and Booth, 1996; Lovell, 1997; Peake, 2004; Robilliard, 1997; Savy, 2004; van Dongen, 2004). These studies dem-onstrate that qualitative theories and method are tolerant to stretch and augmentation, or at least should be, if they are to include all conditions of human life.

Further, I suggested that nurses speak from the moral standpoints provided by Frank's (1995) concepts of *witness* and *duty*. I outlined and exemplified Hyden's (1997) three narra-tive types to show their utility for speaking for very impaired sufferers. I proposed that unruly empirical material be under-stood as *liminal narrativity* that awaits creative interpretation so that it may be conveyed in its own ambiguous terms. At the same time, I suggested cautious use of typologies and cat-egories that press *liminal narrativity* into their service. The means of speaking about dementing illness and speaking for very ill sufferers should, as Frank (1995, p.138) puts it, leave listeners and readers 'conscious of remaining on the edge of a silence ... gazing at what remains in excess of the analyzable'.

Note

1. I use the term sufferer and its relative, patient, aware that suffer-ing, as medically defined in terms of physical and mental pain, is not easy to determine. However, following Kleinman (1995), I define suffering as an integral dimension of human life, an experiential outcome of events such as illness that constrain lived experience.

References

Adams T., 'Kitwood's approach to dementia and dementia care: A critical but appreciative review', *Journal of Advanced Nursing*, 23: 5 (1996) 948–953.

Anderson M., 'To many Katy was just a silhouette', *Journal of Gerontological Nursing*, 12: 2 (1986) 48.

Bender M., and R. Cheston, 'Inhabitants of a lost kingdom: A model of the subjective experiences of dementia', *Ageing and Society*, 17 (1997) 513–532.

Blum N., 'The management of stigma by Alzheimer family care-givers', *Journal of Contemporary Ethnography*, 20: 3 (1991) 263–284.

Blumer H., *Symbolic Interactionism: Perspective and Method* (Berkeley: University of California Press, 1969).

Bogdan R., and S. Taylor, 'Toward a sociology of acceptance: the other side of the study of deviance', *Social Policy*, 18 (1987) 34–39.

Bohling H., 'Communication with Alzheimers' patients: An analysis of caregiver listener patterns', *Journal of Aging and Human Development*, 33: 4 (1991) 249–267.

Booth T., and W. Booth, 'Sounds of silence: Narrative research with inarticulate subjects', *Disability and Society*, 11: 1 (1996) 55–69.

Bruner E., 'Experience and its expressions', in V. Turner and E. Bruner (eds), *The Anthropology of Experience* (Urbana: University of Illinois Press, 1986).

Bruner J., *Making Stories: Law, Literature and Life* (New York: Farrar, Strauss, and Giroux, 2002).

Cheston R., 'Stories and metaphors: Talking about the past in a psychotherapy group for people with dementia', *Ageing and Society*, 16 (1996) 579–602.

Cohen D., 'The subjective experience of Alzheimer's disease: The anatomy of an illness as perceived by patients and families', *The American Journal of Alzheimer's Care and Related Disorders and Research*, (May/June 1991) 6–11.

Crisp J., 'Empty ramblings or empowering narratives: The discourse of the Alzheimer's sufferer', *Meridian*, 11: 2 (1992) 48–53.

Crisp J., 'Making sense of the stories that people with Alzheimer's tell: A journey with my mother', *Nursing Inquiry*, 2: 3 (1995) 133–140.

Downs M., 'The emergence of the person in dementia research', *Ageing and Society*, 17 (1996) 597–607.

Estes C., and E. Binney, 'The biomedicalization of aging: Dangers and dilemmas', *The Gerontologist*, 29: 5 (1989) 587–596.

Feil N., *Validation – The Feil Method* (Cleveland: Edward Feil Productions, 1982).

Fontana A., and R. Smith, 'Alzheimer's disease victims: The unbecoming of self and the normalization of competence', *Sociological Perspectives*, 32: 1 (1989) 35–46.

Frank A., 'Can we research suffering?' *Qualitative Health Research*, 11: 3 (2001) 353–362.

Frank A., *The Wounded Storyteller: Body, Illness and Ethics* (Chicago: University of Chicago Press, 1995).

Goffman E., *The Presentation of Self in Everyday Life* (Harmondsworth: Penguin, 1959).

Goffman E., *Stigma: Notes on the Management of Spoiled Identity* (New Jersey: Englewood Cliffs, 1963).

Golander H., and A. Raz, 'The mask of dementia: Images of "demented residents" in a nursing ward', *Ageing and Society*, 16 (1996) 269–285.

Gubrium J., 'Incommunicables and poetic documentation in the Alzheimer's disease experience', *Semiotica*, 72 (1988) 235–253.

Gubrium J., 'The social preservation of mind: The Alzheimer's disease experience', *Symbolic Interaction*, 9: 1 (1986) 37–51.

Gubrium J., and J. Holstein, *The New Language of Qualitative Method* (New York: Oxford University Press, 1997).

Hamilton H., *Conversations with an Alzheimer's Patient: An Interactional Sociolinguistic Study* (Cambridge University Press: Cambridge, 1994).

Harding N., and C. Palfrey, *The Social Construction of Dementia: Confused Professionals* (London: Jessica Kingsley, 1997).

Harris P. and G. Sterin, 'Insider's perspective: defining and preserving the self in dementia', *Journal of Mental Health and Aging*, 5: 3 (1999) 241–256.

Holst G., and I. Hallberg, 'Exploring the meaning of everyday life for those suffering with dementia', *American Journal of Alzheimer's Disease and Other Dementias*, 18: 6 (2003) 359–365.

Hydén L., 'Illness and narrative', *Sociology of Health and Illness*, 19: 1 (1997) 48–69.

Killick J., and C. Cordonnier, *Openings: Dementia Poems and Photographs* (London: Hawker, 2000).

Killick J., and K. Allan, *Communication and the Care of People with Dementia* (Buckingham: Open University Press, 2002).

Kirmayer L., 'Broken narratives: Clinical encounters and the poetics of illness experience', in C. Mattingly and L. Garro (eds), *Narrative and the Cultural Construction of Illness and Healing* (Berkeley: University of California Press, 2000).

Kitwood T., 'The dialectics of dementia with particular reference to Alzheimer's disease', *Ageing and Society*, 10 (1990)177–196.

Kitwood T., 'Towards a theory of dementia care: The interpersonal process', *Ageing and Society*, 13 (1993) 51–61.

Kitwood T., and K. Bredin K, 'Towards a theory of dementia care: Personhood and well-being', *Ageing and Society*, 12 (1992) 269–287.

Kleinman A., *Writing at the Margin: A Discourse between Anthropology and Medicine* (Berkeley: University of California Press, 1995).

Kristeva J., *Powers of Horror: An Essay on Abjection* (New York: Columbia University Press, 1982).

Lovell A., ' "This city is my mother". Narratives of schizophrenia and homelessness', *American Anthropologist*, 99: 2 (1997) 355–368.

Luken P., 'Social identity in later life', *International Journal of Aging and Human Development*, 25: 3 (1987) 177–193.

Lyman K., 'Bringing the social back in: A critique of the biomedicalization of dementia', *The Gerontologist*, 29 (1989) 597–605.

Maas M., E. Swanson, J. Specht, and K. Buckwalter, 'Alzheimer's special care units', *Nursing Clinics of North America*, 29: 1 (1994) 173–191.

Mace N., *Losing a Million Minds: Confronting the Tragedy of Alzheimer's Disease and Other Dementias* (Washington, DC: US Government Printing Office, 1987).

Mead G., *Mind, Self and Society* (Chicago: University of Chicago Press, 1934).

Miesen B., 'Attachment theory and dementia', in G. Jones and B. Miesen (eds), *Care-giving in Dementia: Research and Applications* (London: Routledge, 1992).

Mills M., 'Narrative identity and dementia: A study of emotion and narrative in older people with dementia', *Ageing and Society*, 17, (1997) 673–698.

Monsour N., and S. Robb, 'Wandering behaviour in old age: A psychosocial study', *Social Work*, 27 (1982) 411–416.

Peake S., Changing the Subject: A Sociology of the Enacting Self, Unpublished thesis (University of Melbourne, Australia, 2004).

Phinney A., 'Fluctuating awareness and the breakdown of the illness narrative in dementia', *The International Journal of Social Research and Practice*, 1: 3 (2002) 329–344.

Phinney A., 'Living with dementia: From the patient's perspective', *Journal of Gerontological Nursing*, 24: 6 (1998) 8–15.

Phinney A., and C. Chesla, 'The lived body in dementia', *Journal of Aging Studies*, 17 (2003) 283–299.

Ramanathan-Abbott V., 'Interactional differences in Alzheimer's discourse: An examination of AD speech across two audiences', *Language and Society*, 23 (1994) 31–58.

Robilliard A., 'Communication problems in the intensive care unit', in R. Hertz (ed.), *Reflexivity and Voice* (Thousand Oaks: Sage, 1997).

Sabat S., and R. Harré, 'The construction and deconstruction of self in Alzheimer's disease', *Ageing and Society*, 12 (1992) 443–461.

Savy P., Identity in Dementia: An Ethnographic Study of the Long-Term Experiences of Sufferers in Long-Term Aged Care Settings, Unpublished thesis (La Trobe University: Australia, 2004).

Savy P., 'Suffering in silence: The problem of bestowing meaning on unspeakable illness', paper presented at the European Sociological Association, 3rd Mid-term Conference, Cardiff University, Wales, UK, 4–6 September 2006.

Shifflett P., and R. Blieszner, 'Stigma and Alzheimer's disease: Behavioral consequences for support groups', *The Journal of Applied Gerontology*, 7: 2 (1988) 147–160.

Shoemaker D., 'Problematic behaviour and the Alzheimer patient: Retrospection as a method of understanding and counselling', *The Gerontologist*, 27: 3 (1987) 370–375.

Surr C., 'Preservation of self in people with dementia living in residential care: A socio-biographical approach', *Social Science and Medicine*, 62 (2006) 1720–1730.

van Dongen E., *Worlds of Psychotic People* (New York: Routledge, 2004).

Vittoria A., ' "Our own little language": Naming and the social construction of Alzheimer's disease', *Symbolic Interaction*, 22: 4 (1999) 361–384.

Woods R., 'Discovering the person with Alzheimer's disease', *Aging and Mental Health*, 5: 2 (2001) 7–16.

Yingling P., 'Shells', *Journal of Gerontological Nursing*, 11: 3 (1985) 44.

10 Social perspectives on depression

Ann Mitchell, Elaine Denny and Sarah Earle

Introduction

Recent advances in genetics, neuroscience and pharmacology continue to dominate discussions about mental health problems to the exclusion of approaches which focus on the social determinants of health and illness (Busfield, 2001). However, there is a long tradition of sociological interest in the influence of social and economic factors on the development and distribution of what Mulvany (2001) describes as the 'disorders of the mind'. Recently, there has also been a wider recognition within government policy of the need to address the rise in mental health problems by tackling the wider determinants of health (for example, see DH, 2006).

Depression is now recognized as one of the major causes of ill health world wide (WH0, 2001). It is thought to be far more common than many physical long term conditions such as asthma or diabetes, yet it remains largely ignored or untreated. There is a significant amount of literature (Lewin, 2007; NICE, 2007; Reading and Reynolds, 2001; Wilkinson et al., 1999) that describes, provides explanations and discusses treatment options for those individuals who may be experiencing depression. Yet despite this abundance of information, depression remains largely misunderstood, under-recognized and under-treated. Some of the reasons for not accessing care and treatment could be attributed to the stigmatization of the condition. Halter (2004) argues that the fear of stigmatization often makes people conceal that they may need help. Similarly in a study of patients attending a psychiatric day centre, Teasdale (1987) found that individuals would hide the reasons for their attendance, as they found a label of mental illness stigmatizing. However major attempts are being made by the Department of Health to improve services for those with mental health problems by raising awareness and the profile of the condition within primary care and secondary care services. For example, The National Service Framework for Mental Health (DH, 1999) and the clinical guidelines for the management of depression (NICE, 2007) show clear recognition and commitment to addressing some of the issues relating to depression.

This chapter explores social perspectives on depression. It begins by outlining biomedical and psychosocial explanations for depression. It then offers a sociological critique of the definitions of depression, as well as its assessment and diagnosis. The chapter outlines the role of nurses in the management of depression in primary care and explores the way in which depression affects people from different social groups.

Explanations for depression

Biomedical

The precise cause of depression remains unknown but there are several explanations that have been put forward as to what may cause it. The focus of the biomedical approach, which is one of the most common explanations for acquiring depression, is based on genetic factors and provides evidence that genes may make a contribution to severe forms of depression (Wilkinson et al., 1999). It has been suggested that genes play a role in bipolar depression and that some people may inherit a tendency to the condition. Changes in biochemistry leading to a reduced level of neurotransmitters serotonin and noradrenaline have been put forward as another explanation. However whether it is the low level of the neurotransmitters that causes depression or whether depression causes them to drop is still being debated (Armstrong, 2002).

Psychosocial

There is much debate about the psychosocial explanation of depression. This explanation is associated with multiple life events. Brown and Harris' (1978) classical study has contributed to this debate and has shaped understanding of how social factors such as major life events can precipitate depression. This study focused on working class women – especially those who were lone mothers – and identified four vulnerability factors that predispose this group of women to the risk of depression. These were: loss of their own mother before the age of 11; having three or more children under the age of 14 at home; lack of supportive and confiding relationship; and, lack of employment outside the home. When the opposites of these factors were found to be present, for example the presence of mother after the age of 11, plus a good relationship with a partner, these acted to protect women against depression.

Reading and Reynolds (2001) postulate that social factors associated with poor housing, hardship, unemployment and living in deprivation can invariably lead to depression. The direct effects of poverty, stress and unemployment are therefore commonly thought to be important underlying features in depression.

Although these perspectives dominate the literature and influence the way depression is constructed and treated, there exists a sociological literature that this chapter will utilize in order to challenge dominant assumptions.

Defining depression

Mood disorders, of which depression is one, have always existed since ancient times. Taylor (1994, p. 273), for example, notes that an, 'Egyptian papyrus of 1500BC contains a discourse on old age and says that "the heart grows heavy and remembers not yesterday"'. The Old Testament also records the erratic behaviour of King Saul as his moods fluctuated between elation and depression. The Greek physician Hippocrates also knew the symptoms of depression believing that it resulted from a surplus of black bile and the condition was known as melancholy. The term 'depression' came into use as a single term to describe the disorders of melancholia, neurasthenia and mopish, which by the middle of the nineteenth century were declining in usage (Pilgrim and Bentall, 1999).

From a biomedical perspective depression is broadly defined as a condition that has severe lowering of mood with extreme sadness, loss of interest in the pleasurable side of life and feelings of guilt and low self worth. Wilkinson et al. (1999) perceive it more as a persistent exaggeration of the everyday feelings that accompany sadness plus a disturbance of mood, of variable severity and duration that is frequently recurrent. Millar and Walsh (2000) describe depression as more than being 'sad' or 'feeling down', but as a mood or affective disorder characterized by pervasive low mood, negative thinking and lack of enjoyment of life. Another significant characteristic of depression is that it sometimes presents in the form of physical symptoms, such as pain, fatigue or headaches rather than emotional symptoms (Millar and Walsh, 2000).

Of course for sociologists the whole notion of 'mental illness' is highly contested. The social construction of disease categories can be seen as a form of social control and surveillance which serves to define what comes to be understood as 'normal' or 'abnormal' behaviour. Pilgrim and Rogers (1999) describe five sociological perspectives of mental illness. Firstly, the theory of social causation accepts the biomedical diagnoses of mental illness, but emphasizes the role of social disadvantage, such as poverty in its causation. Secondly, societal reaction, or labelling theory, considers how behaviour deemed abnormal is at first denied or explained (primary deviance) and later, perhaps when a crisis is reached redefined as a mental illness (secondary deviance). Thirdly, and influenced by both Freud and Marx, critical theorists explore the interrelationship between the mind and society in order to explain mental illness, whereas social constructionists view social context as crucial to the construction of a discourse that is conceptualized as mental illness. Finally, critical or social realism accepts the reality of mental illness, but argues that the way it is interpreted and managed is socially and historically specific.

This brief description serves to illustrate the differences between a biomedical perspective which focuses on an individual categorisation of symptoms, and sociological perspectives which critically explore both the concept of mental illness as a category and the role of mental health workers (psychiatrists, nurses, etc.) in its management.

The next section considers the way in which depression is diagnosed and defined medically, and uses a sociological analysis in order to explore some of the problematic issues that are raised.

Assessment and diagnosis of depression

Diagnostic tools

A comprehensive clinical assessment is considered helpful in gaining a full holistic picture of an individual's mental health problem. An assessment that takes into consideration the psychological, social, cultural and physical characteristics of the service user plus the quality of interpersonal relationships that they have engaged in. In order to do this effectively, a range of diagnostic scales or tools are normally used in order to classify, recognize, diagnose or to categorize depression but these can be based on arbitrarily defined symptoms. The classifications generally used within psychiatry include the International Classification of Diseases (ICD 10) (WHO, 1994) and the Diagnostic and Statistical Manual of Mental Disorders (DSM IV) (American Psychiatric Association, 1994). These diagnostic scales aid the practitioner to identify whether the depression is mild, moderate or severe. For the DSM IV (American Psychiatric Association, 1994) depression is diagnosed when five or more of the symptoms occur in the same two week period. A similar principle is used for ICD 10 but four symptoms indicate a mild episode, six a moderate and eight a severe episode. These are complex scales normally used by very experienced mental health practitioners. The DSM IV diagnostic criteria for depression has been assumed to offer the most valid definition and description of the experience of depression. However criticism has been made of these classifications, both conceptually and as diagnostic tools. As a tool Hagen (2007) reports that the DSM IV is ambiguous and that it is left to clinician judgement to decide whether certain behaviours are present in such a way or for such a period of time that constitutes a diagnosis. He further argues that many mental health practitioners simply take the reliability and validity of the DSM IV for granted but closer examination will demonstrate that the DSM IV criteria can allow for several possible different clusters of symptoms, all of which can still meet the diagnostic criteria for depression (Hagen, 2007).

There are, however, more fundamental critiques of classification systems. Kutchins and Kirk (1997) argue that DSM pathologizes everyday behaviour, so that the criteria for depression includes such commonly experienced events such as apathy, sleep disturbance or appetite change, only five of which need to be met for a diagnosis of depression to be conferred. If two of the criteria are met a diagnosis of 'subsyndromal depression' can be made. What the DSM does not do is provide any indication of how to distinguish between pathology and a variation of normal behaviour. Further, Kutchins and Kirk state that there is not a single major study to show that DSM IV is used with high reliability by mental health clinicians.

There are additional scales that can assist in assessing the service user's mental state to confirm their diagnosis. Depression rating scales were developed during the 1950s with the advent of antidepressant drugs (Hagen, 2007). They provided a tool that could be used to test the severity of depression in an individual in order to assess required dosage, and also assess response to the drugs over time. The Beck Depression Inventory (BDI-II), the Hospital Anxiety and Depression (HAD), Geriatric Depression Scale (GDS) and the Edinburgh Post Natal Depression Scale (EPDS) are normally used in primary care due to their ease of use. Beck is one of the most commonly used scales as it is self administered and only requires five to ten minutes to complete. One of its main strengths is its ease of administration, scoring and interpretation of the data. However criticisms have been made concerning the scale in that despite claiming neutrality, it actually reflects a cognitive-behavioural perspective on depression (Hagen, 2007). It is also gender biased and Anglocentric, issues that will be discussed below. According to Hagen (2007) limited nursing literature has critically examined its use within mental health nursing practice.

The GDS and EPDS scales have also been criticized for their validity and reliability. Rating scales reduce very complex behaviour patterns to a linear or 'checklist' inventory, which serves to reify depression. Armstrong (2002) reminds us that no scale should replace the need for a full holistic assessment of the person.

Depression types

Another way of classifying depression is by subdividing the condition into different types (Armstrong, 2002; Wilkinson et al., 1999). Within psychiatry this is labelled as reactive or endogenous depression, bipolar or unipolar, neurotic or psychotic, post natal and seasonal affective disorder. Each type has a long list of specific symptoms or behaviours that can be exhibited. Reactive depression can thus occur in response to a major life event, for example, divorce, or the loss of one's job, and symptoms include worry, anxiety and sleep problems. This type of depression may only require treatment if the symptoms persists. Endogenous depression implies that the depression occurs from within and symptoms range from sleep disturbance, loss of concentration and memory and responds to antidepressants. Bipolar depression, also known as manic depressive psychosis, presents with mood swings with periods of elation followed by depressive episodes. This is very serious and enduring illness that has a high rate of reoccurrence. Unipolar depression is defined as depression without mood swings and is normally perceived as a recurrent depression.

Further classification used is to differentiate between neurotic and psychotic depression where neurotic depression is the least 'serious' of the two. Neurotic depression is perceived as a preoccupation with an emotional trauma that precedes the illness, for example loss of an ideal or loved one. This type of depression has no psychotic features whereas psychotic depression features a series of delusions and hallucinations. Dysthymia is a chronic mild depression defined by the presence of depressive symptoms for at least two years. A diagnosis is made when the symptoms are not present for the majority of time but may come and go for a few days at a time (Armstrong, 2002).

Postnatal depression (or postnatal mental illness) is another type of mental health problem that has similar symptoms to depression but normally occurs after the birth of a baby (Armstrong, 2002). It may start as 'baby blues' which is usually mild with tearfulness and occurs in the first ten days following the birth. It is usually perceived as a 'normal' reaction to motherhood but is of short duration and prognosis is good. This emotional feeling can then lead to a depressive episode. Noble (2005) suggests that 25 per cent of those affected by the baby blues experience post natal depression. Puerperal psychosis is a more serious psychotic disorder after the onset of which usually occurs several weeks after childbirth; it is characteriszd by symptoms such as hallucinations, delusions and inappropriate behaviour. Onset is quick but inpatient care is offered to mother and baby and prognosis is good.

Research into post natal depression by Morgan et al. (1991) has demonstrated that what is considered to be normal life events for women have been submitted to a process of distortion by the medical profession. Their increasing interference has led to professional dominance of the condition. However a more recent study by Hanley and Long (2006, p. 155) have questioned whether 'postnatal depression justifies its medical definition or whether it is socially constructed'. The findings from this small scale study have shown to 'some extent that postnatal depression is a consequence of social deterioration rather than a purely physical reaction to motherhood' and that further work may be necessary to understand the experiences of women with this condition.

The types of depression discussed so far are constantly being reviewed and updated but what can be gleaned from these descriptions is that individuals exhibit different symptoms, so this account demonstrates that complexities of human behaviour are defined mainly by assessing biological symptoms. This reductionist approach relies heavily on a biomedical model of assessment by looking for categories and symptoms rather than concentrating on the other facets of the individual's life in order to gain a full holistic picture of what is happening to them. In western societies emotional or psychological differences have become increasingly medicalized. What should be captured are the individual psychological and social responses to any given situation, which are often neglected (Hanley and Long, 2006). Pilgrim and Bentall (1999, p. 271) point to the ambiguity about what constitutes depression arguing that 'the contemporary western notion of "depression" is confused, woolly and inadequate as a basis for formulating mental health problems.' Writing from a critical realist perspective they warn against accepting the dualistic ideas of the biomedical model and social constructionism, and suggest a third way that recognizes the reality of misery and its determinants without following the naïve reality of a psychiatric notion of 'depression' as an acultural and ahistoric medical category.

Addressing depression in primary care

One of the most common mental health problems seen in primary care is depression. Statistics suggest that one person in five is currently depressed and up to one in three will experience depression at some point in their lives (Effective Health Care Bulletin, 2002). Yet even with this high incidence, it is often perceived by some as being a trivial condition that does not necessarily require medical attention. Unfortunately it is often misdiagnosed or not treated due to failure by the General Practitioner (GP) in not recognizing the symptoms that the person may be exhibiting. The focus of a consultation with the GP may be on the physical manifestation of the condition rather than trying to get to the root of the service user's problem. GPs' consultations tend to be brief so vital signs are often missed in order to keep to the allocated time slot. That said, diagnozing depression is not an easy task within primary care because there are varying degrees of this condition which range from feeling sad or unhappy to experiencing severe symptoms. At the most severe end of this range, the feeling of hopelessness can sometimes lead to either suicidal attempts or suicide (MacDonald, 2004).

Other members of the Primary Care Team, particularly practice nurses, can play an important role in recognizing the symptoms of depression. Practice nurses are becoming more involved in the diagnosis, monitoring and management of depression (Lewin, 2007) but training is essential for them in order to recognize and monitor symptoms. Assessing the severity of depression can be particularly difficult for the primary care team especially if they do not have the necessary skills and expertise to do so. Nurses in primary care who have received training can provide support for the service user with milder forms of depression. MacDonald (2004) notes that:

> experienced practice nurses will feel better able to identify with those suffering from the milder forms of depression. As an empathic listener they can give valuable support to those who may feel terrible but know at some level they will come out of it. They are able to function in society and depression may make sense in the context of their life. (MacDonald, 2004, p. 2)

When severe or negative enduring symptoms of depression persist, health care practitioners in primary care may not have the necessary skills and expertise to respond to service users so referral to secondary care services might be required. Secondary mental health practitioners now provide a range of services in the community and in inpatient units. Inpatient facilities have changed over the years from the rather large Victorian hospitals that were tucked away from the rest of the community to more 'discrete' customized units. These generally accommodate service users with a broad spectrum of mental health needs. Crisis resolution and home treatment teams have been developed for service users with severe depression who present as a serious risk. Prognosis very much depends on the type and severity of the individual's depression However, depression can be treated successfully although recurrence is common for some forms of depression.

Many people find it difficult to imagine what it would be like to have a mental health problem and even when they experience a common mental health problem like depression, they may keep it a secret from family, friends and their health care practitioner (Armstrong, 2002). Even when they recognize that something is wrong, they may call it a 'nervous breakdown' or just 'nerves'. The fear of being labelled may prevent them from revealing what is happening to them because, for some people, mental illness is shrouded in secrecy, fear and ignorance. Stigma affects all groups in society and is often perceived as another barrier to seeking help for a depressive condition (Mitchell, 2002). Halter (2004) conducted a small scale study in America and highlights that the fear of stigmatization often prevents people from seeking help because they perceive themselves as being weak. Additionally: 'They are unaware of what kind of help they need, don't know where help is available and are uncertain that there would be any benefit to seeking help' (Halter, 2004, p. 178). Further studies (Byrne, 2000; Huxley, 1993) have shown that there is no doubt that negative attitudes to mental health problems across a range of groups living in the community do exist. Research by Barrio (2000) has also shown that minority ethnic groups are even more affected by stigma and that they are more likely to either keep their mental health problem to themselves or within the family.

The impact of depression on different social groups

Depression in older people

Many older people are vulnerable to depression and it is the most common mental health problem to affect them. Indeed it is often seen as an 'inevitable' part of the ageing process. The clinical features of this condition are the same in this group as in younger people however presentation may differ and diagnosis may be more difficult due to symptoms of physical illnesses. In some instances, depression may also be masked by dementia. Depression and dementia share many similar symptoms so it can be difficult to distinguish between the two illnesses when people present with either of them (Wright and Persad, 2007).

Even though older people visit their GP twice as often as younger people, their depression is less likely to be recognized or treated. A large study in primary care (Crawford et al., 1998) highlighted that only 38 per cent of older people with a diagnosis for depression had received any treatment or referral. Older people my also fail to recognize that they have depression and may articulate their feelings with reference to physical symptoms such as tiredness and light headed feelings. Murray et al. (2006) observed that older people typically present with somatic rather than psychological complaints and are likely to become depressed after a physical illness. They are less likely to come in and say that they are depressed when in consultation with their GP hence the reason why the depression may be misdiagnosed. The key findings of Murray et al.'s (2006) study indicate that older people are reluctant to acknowledge depression because they do not regard psychological distress as a medical problem or sufficiently important to take up GPs time. They believe that admitting feelings of depression is a sign of weakness and that depression carries stigma.

For sociologists, ageism plays an important part in the way in which depression and other mental health problems are managed in the older population. Chambers (2005), drawing on the work of social gerontologists, defines ageism as the following:

- marginalization
- the use of dismissive and demeaning language
- humour and mockery
- physical, sexual, emotional and financial abuse
- economic disadvantage
- and, restricted opportunities or life chances (Chambers, 2005, p. 112)

As a result of living in an ageist society, Chambers argues, older people often internalize ageist views. Furthermore, Bernard (1998) suggests that ageism is not only evident in the general population but it also rife among those who care for older people in a professional capacity, including nurses. There is, however, a large body of evidence that places the nurse-patient relationship at the heart of mental health nursing (for example, see Dowling, 2006 and Silverstein, 2006). Indeed, it could be argued that an effective nurse-patient relationship is a central feature for the successful management of all long term conditions.

Gender and depression

There is much documented evidence (Nazroo et al., 1998; Ramsay et al., 2001) regarding gender differences and mental health problems. The following quote from the World Health Organization aptly describes the differences between women and men:

> Research shows that socially constructed differences between women and men in roles and responsibilities, status and power interact with biological differences between the sexes and contribute to the differences in the nature of mental health problems suffered. (WHO, 2002, p. 2)

This explanation highlights that certain factors may play a key role in how these two groups may articulate their mental health problems and, in this context, depression. Genetic and biological factors have been shown to predispose more women to depression that men (WHO, 2002), the reason being that as a part of the menstrual cycle mood swings can occur due to hormonal changes and psychological distress associated with the reproductive health system. However there is limited research that has studied men's reproductive functioning in relation to their mental health, and single men are also overrepresented in statistics on depression (Prior, 1999). It is questionable whether comparisons can be made between men and women. The BDI has also been held to bias a diagnosis of depression in favour of women (Hagen, 2007). Women score higher than men on the scale, but it has been accused of gender bias in the use of terms such as 'crying' that may hold different meanings for men and for women. Hagen further argues that in using the DSM IV twice as many women as men are diagnosed with depression, yet the part played by contextual factors, such as gender discrimination or higher rates of sexual abuse are rarely considered. Prior (1999) also points to intolerable constraints in the traditional female role as an important factor in the development of depression in women. Female scholars have also been critical of DSM IV, arguing that the categories within it reflect the values of expert panels comprising mainly of middle class white men (for example, see Kutchins and Kirk, 1997).

It is widely documented that women present to their GPs more frequently with physical and psychological complaints as opposed to men who seek help much later when they have a problem (Johnson and Buszewicz, 1996). As a consequence there may be more statistical information about women seeking help but that does not necessarily mean that they have more episodes of depression. Research suggests that men may find it difficult to express emotional distress and will present later to their GP but are more likely to be referred to secondary care services than are women (WHO, 2002). However, Nazroo et al. (1998, p. 326) are rather dismissive of such research and provide some evidence in their study that 'the main gender differences in depression are largely as a result of differences in roles and the stresses and expectations that go with them'. Therefore in trying to assess whether they are valid differences between women and men with regard to depression, more research is needed.

Ethnicity and depression

Culture also plays an important part in defining an individual's response to mental health problems but this response can be open to misinterpretation. Ahmed and Bhugra suggest that:

> ...culture can influence depression in a variety of ways, and cultural differences will translate into distinct manifestations and treatment expectations of the illness. Discrepancies in the understanding and conceptual beliefs of depressive illness between patient and doctor, the complicated effects of acculturation, and various culture-specific psychosocial factors result in confusion in the understanding of the illness. (Ahmed and Bhugra, 2006, p. 417)

Despite this much research on the mental health of Black and Minority Ethnic (BME) groups has focused on just two of these groups – African-Caribbean and South Asian people. Iley and Nazroo (2001) state that if we look at treatment statistics, rates of depression for African-Caribbean people are much lower, and for South Asians slightly lower than for white people. This does not necessarily reflect incidence, however, as the community based Fourth National Survey of Ethnic Minorities reported higher levels for both groups (cited in Iley and Nazroo, 2001). In order to explain these discrepancies is it perhaps useful to consider the way people interpret and respond to symptoms of depression. People from BME groups are especially likely to present with physical symptoms when they are depressed. As Ahmed and Bhugra (2006) have highlighted they may present with somatic symptoms and use their 'culturally determined idioms of distress to express how they are experiencing illness'. They argue that in order to make an accurate diagnosis, current diagnostic criteria should be supplemented with an approach that incorporates somatic symptoms. Fernando (2002) further argues that depression – as it is understood in psychiatric circles – should be regarded as a 'western disease':

> Taking the alleged reports that 'depression' in non-European cultures is characterised by somatic symptoms rather than psychic ones...a psychologically depression is different from one associated with somatic experience. (Fernando, 2002, p. 130)

Some researchers argue that people from minority ethnic groups are less likely to seek professional treatment for depression (Mallinson and Popay, 2007). It has also been suggested that primary care practitioners may not always be responsive to the needs of BME groups because of differences in expectations. These differences may occur because of the individual's interpretation of their symptoms of depression which may be entirely different to that of the primary care practitioner. Other reasons suggested why ethnic minority groups may not seek support or treatment for their depression have either been associated with the lack of recognition of the clinical symptoms of depression or that they do not have the language to describe what is happening to them. However, Mallinson and Popay (2007, p. 858) have identified studies that 'challenged this generalisation'. In particular, they refer to the study of Fenton and Sadiq-Sangster (1996) which noted that 'there are commonalities in the experience of depression and anxiety across ethnic groups in terms of feelings, thoughts and symptoms. These may be described differently and responses might also differ but this does not mean that people are unable to recognise psychic symptoms'.

However what should be considered is that members from these BME groups who present with a depressive illness should not be perceived as just one homogenous group. Instead, each discrete grouping may have has its own beliefs of what is depression and this may shape their help seeking behaviour and response to treatment.

The experience of mental illness in Irish immigrants to the United Kingdom demonstrates that factors other than colour also need to be considered when attempting to explain mental illness and BME groups. Rates of hospital admission for depression in people of Irish descent who are living in England are much higher than for those born in England, and for BME groups (Pilgrim and Rogers, 1999). This is thought to be the result of two factors, material deprivation (e.g., poverty, forced migration, and colonial suppression) and cultural practices (e.g., sexual repression, female subordination and strict approaches to childrearing).

Conclusion

Biomedical explanations dominate contemporary understandings, diagnoses and treatment for depression. However, social perspectives offer a critical viewpoint. Some perspectives highlight the role of socio-economic disadvantage as a cause of depression, whereas others focus on the social construction of mental health problems and identify the social context as crucial to the construction of certain feelings and behaviours as 'abnormal'. Within the context of health service provision, researchers have usefully explored the ways in which mental health problems come to be diagnosed and treated, showing that there are marked differences, for example, between women and men, as well as between people from different ethnic groups. There is an important role to be played by nurses, and other health care practitioners in the diagnosis, treatment and management of depression particularly within the context of an increasingly over-burdened health service. Writing specifically about the role of nurses within primary care, Mead, Bower and Gask (1997) have argued that whilst the routine mental health work that nurses perform should be better recognized, there is a need for increased education and training opportunities for nurses to enable them to support people with depression.

References

Ahmed K., and D. Bhugra, 'Diagnosis and management of depression across cultures', *Psychiatry*, 5: 11 (2006) 417–419.

American Psychiatric Association, *DSM-IV Diagnostic and Statistical Manual of Disorders*, 4th edn (Washington DC: American Psychiatric Association, 1994).

Armstrong, E. *A Guide to Mental Health for Nurses in Primary Care* (Oxford: Radcliffe Medical Press, 2002).

Barrio C., 'The cultural relevance of community support programs', *Psychiatric Services*, 51 (2000) 879–884.

Bernard M., 'Backs to the future? Reflections on women, ageing and nursing', *Journal of Advanced Nursing*, 27: 3 (1998) 633–640.

Brown G.W., and T.O. Harris, *Social Origins of Depression* (London: Tavistock, 1978).

Busfield J. (ed.), *Rethinking the Sociology of Mental Health* (Oxford: Blackwell Publishers, 2001).

Byrne P., 'Stigma of mental illness and ways of diminishing it', *Advances in Psychiatric Treatment*, 6 (2000) 65–72.

Chambers P., 'Contemporary perspectives on ageing', in E. Denny and S. Earle (eds) *Sociology for Nurses* (Cambridge: Polity, 2005).

Crawford M.J., M. Prince, P. Menezes and A.H. Mann, 'The recognition and treatment of depression in older people in primary care', *International Journal of Geriatric Psychiatry*, 13: 3 (1998) 172–176.

Department of Health (DH) *National Service Framework for Mental Health* (London: The Stationery Office, 1999).

Department of Health (DH) *Choosing Health: Supporting the Physical Health Needs of People with Severe Mental Illness* (London: The Stationery Office, 2006).

Dowling M., 'The sociology of intimacy in the nurse-patient relationship', *Nursing Standard*, 20: 23 (2006) 48–55.

Effective Health Care Bulletin, *Improving the Recognition and Management of Depression in Primary Care*, 7: 5 (2002) 9.

Fenton S., and Sadiq-Sangster, 'Culture, relativism and the expression of mental distress: South Asian women in Britain', *Sociology of Health and Illness*, 18: 1 (1996) 66–85.

Fernando S., *Mental Health, Race and Culture*, Second Edition (Hampshire: Palgrave, 2002).

Hagen B., 'Measuring melancholy: A critique of the Beck Depressive Inventory and its use in mental health nursing', *International Journal of Mental Health Nursing*, 16: 2 (2007) 108–115.

Halter J., 'The stigma of seeking care and depression', *Archives of Psychiatric Nursing*, XVIII5:(2004) 178–184.

Hanley J., and B. Long, 'A study of Welsh mothers' experiences of postnatal depression', *Midwifery*, 22: 2 (2006) 147–157.

Huxley P., 'Location stigma. A survey of community attitudes to mental illness: Enlightment and stigma', *Journal of Mental Health*, 2 (1993) 73–80.

Johnson S., M. Buszewicz. 'Women's mental illness', in K. Abel, M. Buszewiz , S. Davison, S. Johnson and E. Staples (eds) *Planning Community Mental Health Services for Women, a Multi-Professional Handbook* (London: Routledge, 1996).

Iley K., and J. Nazroo, 'Ethnic inequalities in mental health', in L. Culley and S. Dyson (eds) *Ethnicity and Nursing Practice* (Basingstoke: Palgrave, 2001).

Kutchins H., and S.A. Kirk, *Driving Us Crazy: DSM – the Psychiatric Bible and the Creation of Mental Disorders* (London: Constable, 1997).

Lewin K., 'Depression assessment', *Practice Nurse*, January 29, 33: 12 (2007) 43–45.

MacDonald P., 'The depressed patient', *Practice Nurse*, October 29, 28: 7 (2004) 17–22.

Mallinson S., and J. Popay, 'Describing depression: ethnicity and the use of somatic imagery accounts of mental illness', *Sociology of Health and Illness*, 29: 6 (2007) 857–871.

Mead N., P. Bower and L. Gask, 'Emotional problems in primary care: what is the potential for increasing the role of nurses?', *Journal of Advanced Nursing*, 26: 5 (1997) 879–890.

Millar E., and M. Walsh, *Mental Health Matters* (Cheltenham: Stanley Thornes, 2000).

Mitchell A., 'Stigma: discrimination, ethnicity and gender issues in primary care', in L. Armstrong (ed.), *The Guide to Mental Health for Nurses in Primary Care* (Abingdon: Radcliffe, 2002).

Morgan M., M. Calnan and N. Manning, *Sociological Approaches to Health and Medicine* (London: Routledge, 1991).

Mulvany J., 'Disability, impairment or illness? The relevance of the social model of disability to the study of mental disorder', in J. Busfield (ed.), *Rethinking the Sociology of Mental Health* (Oxford: Blackwell Publishers, 2001).

Murray J., S. Banerjee, R. Byng, A. Tylee, D. Bhugra and A. Macdonald, 'Primary care professionals' perceptions of depression in older people: a qualitative study', *Social Science and Medicine*, 63: 5 (2006) 1363–1373.

National Institute for Health and Clinical Excellence (NICE), *Depression: Management of Depression in Primary and Secondary Care* (London, NICE, 2007).

Noble R.E., 'Depression in women', *Metabolism*, 54: 5, Supplement 1 (2005) 49–52.

Nazroo J.Y., A.C. Edwards and G.W. Brown, 'Gender differences in the prevalence of depression: artefact, alternative disorders, biology or role?', *Sociology of Health and Illness*, 20: 3 (1998) 312–330.

Pilgrim D., and R. Bentall, 'The medicalisation of misery: A critical realist analysis of the concept of depression', *Journal of Mental Health* 8: 3 (1999) 261–274.

Pilgrim D., and A. Rogers, *A Sociology of Mental Health and Illness* (Buckingham: Open University Press, 1999).

Prior P.M., *Gender and Mental Health* (Basingstoke: Macmillan, 1999).

Ramsay R., S. Welch and E. Youard, 'Needs of women patients with mental illness', *Advances in Psychiatric Treatment*, 7 (2001) 85–92.

Reading R., and S. Reynolds, 'Debt, social disadvantage and maternal depression', *Social Science and Medicine*, 53: 4 (2001) 441–453.

Rogers A., and D. Pilgrim, *Mental Health and Inequality* (Basingstoke: Palgrave Macmillan, 2003).

Silverstein C.M., 'Therapeutic interpersonal interactions: the sacrificial lamb?', *Perspectives in Psychiatric Care*, 42: 1 (2006) 33–42.

Taylor C.M., *Essentials of Psychiatric Nursing*, 14 edn (Missouri: Mosby, 1994).

Teasdale K., 'Stigma and psychiatric day care', *Journal of Advanced Nursing*, 12 (1987) 339–346.

World Health Organization (WHO) *ICD-10, Classifications of Mental and Behavioural Disorders* (Geneva: WHO, 1994).

World Health Organization (WHO) *Gender and Mental Health* (Geneva: WHO, 2002).

World Health Organization Regional Office for Europe (WHO) *Mental Health in Europe – Stop Exclusion, Dare to Care. World Mental Health Day* (Copenhagen: WHO Regional Office for Europe, 2001).

Wilkinson G., B. Moore and P. Moore, *Treating People with Depression* (Abingdon: Radcliffe Medical Press, 1999).

Wright S.L., C. Persad, 'Distinguishing between depression and dementia in older persons: neuropsychological and neuropathological correlates', *Journal of Geriatric Psychiatry & Neurology*, 20: 4 (2007) 189–198.

11 Obesity: a long term condition?

Sarah Earle

Introduction: The obesity pandemic

Over the last 30 or 40 years, the prevalence of obesity and overweight has increased to, what could be described as, pandemic proportions. Globally, there are more than one billion overweight adults, 300 million of whom are obese (WHO, 2003). According to official figures, in Europe – and in the United States – the majority of adults are overweight or obese and England, Wales and Scotland have relatively high rates of obesity in comparison to most other countries in Europe (House of Commons Health Committee, 2004). Global rates of childhood obesity have also increased. Worldwide, there are now 177 million school-age children who are overweight or obese. In the United Kingdom, childhood obesity and overweight has increased significantly since the 1980s. For example, figures published in 2005 indicate that 22 per cent of boys and 28 per cent of girls aged 2 to 15 in the United Kingdom were either overweight or obese (BMA, 2005).

As is the case with most other long term conditions, obesity is increasingly common in societies characterized by industrialization, affluence and wealth. It is now a major contributor to the global burden of disease, accounting for between 2 and 7 per cent of total health care costs. In England, a conservative estimate of the total cost of obesity – which includes both direct and indirect costs – is thought to be well over 3 billion pounds (House of Commons Health Committee, 2004). However, the classification and measurement of obesity are not unproblematic and many social scientists question the very concept of an obesity pandemic. This chapter begins within a discussion of obesity and its associated co-morbidities, offering a sociological critique of the classification and measurement of obesity and overweight. Next, drawing on feminist sociology, disability politics, and on the sociological concepts of stigma and metaphor this chapter explores sociological and social science understandings of obesity and reflects on the meaning and representation of obesity and overweight within society. Finally, the chapter considers the role of health care and the role of nurses in particular, in the prevention and treatment of obesity and overweight.

Obesity and the risk to public health

Obesity: the 'disease'

Sociologists are interested in how and why certain physical (and mental) states come to be defined as a medical condition. Zola (1973, p. 261) argues that, 'if anything can be shown in some way to affect the workings of the body and to a lesser extent the mind, then it can be labelled ... "a medical problem"'. In other words, sociologists argue that what comes to be defined as a disease is dependent upon a range of political and economic factors, rather than solely on scientific, clinical or medical ones. For example, writing about the construction of the menopause as an 'oestrogen-deficiency' disease in the 1960s, Hunt (1994) and Lee (1998) both argue that this was strongly associated with the development, and increasing availability and marketing, of hormone replacement therapies rather than with the recognition of oestrogen deficiency, which had occurred much before this time.

Writing specifically about obesity, Conway and Rene (2004) argue that the classification of obesity is complex and has been influenced by a range of values, as well as by politics, economics, science and semantics. Obesity only first became classified as a disease in 1985. However, even today, its classification is disputed. Gard and Wright (2005) suggest that obesity is not actually a disease, but simply a risk factor for other diseases (such as diabetes). They suggest that: 'Calling obesity a disease because obesity is associated with various non-communicable diseases is like identifying short men as ill because of the established association between short stature and ischaemic heart disease' (Gard and Wright 2005, p. 95).

Other commentators highlight the similarity of obesity to medical conditions such as hypertension, for example by pointing out that not all people who are obese or overweight are ill – and indeed some are extremely fit and healthy – just as some people who are normal weight are healthy, whereas others are ill.

Although the classification of obesity is disputed, adults who are overweight or obese seem to be at a greater risk of a range of co-morbidities such as type 2 diabetes, cardiovascular disease, stroke and certain types of cancer (e.g., cancer of the colon) (WHO, 2003). Metabolic syndrome (whose classification is also contested), which denotes a cluster of conditions including high blood pressure, raised blood sugar and cholesterol levels, together with abdominal obesity, is also believed to significantly increase the risk of cardiovascular disease and type 2 diabetes (BMA, 2005). Indeed the term 'diabesity' is now commonly used to reflect the greatly increased risk of diabetes for people who are obese. In children, similar patterns of co-morbidity are evident. For example, more young children are presenting with the early symptoms of metabolic syndrome. Type 2 diabetes (which has always most commonly been found in adults) is now also increasingly being seen in children. The early onset of diabetes is alarming since this increases the risk of complications – such as visual impairment, kidney failure and peripheral vascular disease – in later life. Given the range of co-morbidities, and the cost of these to individuals and to society, the prevention and treatment of obesity is paramount; key to this is the measurement and surveillance of obesity and overweight in populations. However, as the next section in this chapter shows, the measurement of obesity is not unproblematic.

Measuring obesity

Given the importance of treating and preventing obesity within populations, the measurement of obesity and overweight in individuals and across populations is of paramount importance. Epidemiological research on obesity relies on reliable systems of classification and measurement. However, as the previous section has highlighted, the classification of obesity is contested and although this disease is widely recognized as one of the biggest unmet public health crises of the twenty-first century there is little consensus on how obesity should be measured. Most commonly, obesity is measured using Body Mass Index (BMI), which is defined as weight in kilograms divided by height in metres squared (kg/m^2). According to this measurement, people with a BMI over 25 kg/m^2 are defined as overweight, whereas those with a BMI of 30 kg/m^2 or over are defined as obese (WHO, 2000). Other anthropometric measurements can also be used to determine obesity. For example, lean body mass can be determined by measuring skinfold thickness. Waist circumference is also seen as a good measure which correlates closely to BMI, and the ratio of waist-to-hip circumference is seen a good approximate index of both intra-abdominal fat and total body fat (or central obesity). Increases in waist circumference also closely correlate to increased risk for various chronic conditions (WHO, 2003).

However, anthropometry is not without its critics particularly when applied to the individual, rather than across populations. Indeed Gard and Wright (2005, p. 94) suggest that much caution is needed if 'science fiction' is not to be represented as 'science fact'. However, even at the level of health surveillance in populations, creating a universal classification system for obesity is problematic for both children and adults, particularly given the ethnically diverse world-population. For example, techniques used to measure body fat have been validated largely on Caucasian populations and, hence, given the differences between ethnic groups may not be valid for non-Caucasian populations (Duerenberg and Duerenberg-Yap, 2001). These ethnic differences are evident in terms of both body fat distribution and in relation to the correlation between percentage body fat and disease risk (Neovius et al., 2004). In a study of BMI and percentage body fat in different adult population groups of Asians, Deurenberg, Deurenberg-Yap and Guricci (2002) found that Asians had higher percentage body fat at lower BMI compared to Caucasians. So, this means that for comparisons of obesity prevalence between ethnic groups, universal BMI cut-off points are inappropriate and different ones should be used. The same study also found considerable differences between Asian groups, for example between Chinese and Indonesians, but also between ethnic groups living in different locations – for example, Chinese groups living in either New York, Beijing or Hong Kong.

Given the rising prevalence of obesity amongst children and associated co-morbidities, such as diabetes, the measurement of childhood obesity, and obesity prevention for children is also important. However, there is currently no universally accepted system for the classification of childhood obesity, although several BMI-based systems are available including that of the WHO and the International Obesity Taskforce (IOTF). Neovius et al. (2004) identify several problems with the use of BMI as an indicator of obesity in childhood and adolescence, some of these are listed in Box 11.1 It is interesting to note that the government white paper in England, *Choosing Health* (DH, 2004), pledged to reintroduce the school medical; the annual weighing and measuring of children in primary schools. However the Royal College of Nursing (RCN), amongst others, opposed this measure. For example, in a newspaper report, John Thain, the RCN advisor on children and young people states:

> We already know that children with weight problems can have low-self esteem. If they are told that the whole class is going to be weighed, how will that make them feel? Children have the right to receive support and advice and not to be singled out...children are going to perceive adults as figures who put them under surveillance. (Quoted in Templeton, 2005, July 17, p. 5)

Box 11.1 Problems associated with BMI measurement in childhood and adolescence

- Increases in BMI during childhood growth are mainly attributable to increases in lean body mass, especially in boys
- The relationship between BMI, fatness and risk is not identical across ethnic groups
- Validity studies using BMI to identify children with excess adiposity have generally documented low to moderate sensitivities for BMI
- The relationship between BMI and fatness may not be stable over time

Source: Adapted from Neovius, 2004, p. 106.

Sociological and social science understandings of obesity

The biomedical classification of obesity and epidemiological approaches to obesity and overweight continue to dominate the obesity agenda to the exclusion of other approaches. Biomedical and epidemiological perspectives influence how obesity is classified and measured as well as how it is experienced and represented, but sociological and social science approaches can also contribute to an understanding of obesity within a social context.

Some social science research has focused on the experience of obesity and overweight on health and psychological well-being. For example, a number of studies indicate that obesity can lead to conditions such as depression in both adults and children (Sjoberg, Nilsson and Leppert, 2005; Heo et al., 2006) as well as a poorer quality of life (Brownell, 2005). Other research studies suggest that obese and overweight people feel that they are discriminated against in employment and education, as well is in other aspects of their daily lives (Carr and Friedman, 2005). However, not all research concurs with this perspective. For example, Wardle and Cooke (2005) suggest that studies typically report poorer psychological well-being amongst people who seek treatment, and that this may not necessarily hold true for the general population. They also argue that obese children are unlikely to be depressed. Similarly, in a study of over 9,000 obese and overweight adults, Doll, Peterson and Stewart-Brown (2000) found that obese people did not experience a deterioration of psychological well-being as a result of obesity or overweight and that such findings in other studies could be explained with reference to the co-morbidities associated with obesity, rather than to obesity itself. Davidson and Knafl (2006), however, warn against the use of biomedical and epidemiological approaches to obesity, arguing that whilst health-care professionals and many researchers typically adopt these approaches, there is no reason to believe that these are shared by others. They argue that, 'This gap between scientific and lay understandings of obesity has led to growing recognition of the need to place the concept in a socio-cultural context' (Davidson and Knafl, 2006, p. 343).

Beginning with the standpoint that the 'personal is polit-ical', feminist writers have also explored the issue of obesity and overweight. Drawing on the concept of patriarchal power (the oppression of women in a society that is dominated by male power) Bordo (1995) suggests that culture maintains a firm hold on women's bodies by defining fatness as 'bad' and thin-ness as 'good'. Writing from a feminist psychological perspec-tive, Chernin (1981) and Orbach (1988) have also expressed concerns with the prevalence of eating disorders amongst women and girls, suggesting that women become damaged by living in a patriarchal society which places unrealistic expect-ations on achieving the 'perfect' body size, shape and weight. It is also worth pointing out that this 'tyranny of slenderness' has meant that, until recently, women in particular have been the primary consumers of a multi-million pound global indus-try that peddles diet foods, books and clubs. Whilst not all commentators agree with feminist perspectives on obesity and overweight, these perspectives have been influential in shaping social science understandings (Gard and Wright, 2005).

Writing critically of feminist perspectives, Cooper (1997) – who defines herself as an 'able-bodied fat woman' – has chosen to define obesity (or fatness) as a disability. She argues that feminism has consistently defined all fat people as either suf-ferers of eating disorders, or as primordial goddesses. Drawing on a social model of disability Cooper identifies the similar-ities between disabled people and fat people, and between dis-ability politics and fat politics, arguing:

> The bodies of fat and disabled people share low social status...Like people with mobility impairments, many fat people are disabled by a lack of access in the physical environment, for example, clothes don't fit, seats are too small, turnstiles are impossible to navigate. Fat and disabled people encounter discrimination in all areas of our lives...where we are constantly reminded that something is wrong with us. Most blatantly congruent are our experiences of medicalisa-tion...When we conceptualise fatness as a disease, we also assume that somehow it must be cured in order for our bodies to function normally. (Cooper, 1997, pp. 36–37)

More recently, attention has also turned to understanding obesity in men. For example, drawing on an ethnographic study of men, masculinities and weight, Monaghan (2007a) suggests that 'while fat has been described as a feminist issue ... it is also being very publicly defined as a worrying masculine issue – with masculinity associated with frailty, vulnerability and increased health risk' (p. 585). Monaghan (2007a, 2007b) also suggests that some men are being damaged by the 'war on obesity' that is waged by healthcare professionals, health agencies, slimming clubs and others, and argues that it is important to reflect on the notion of 'fatness' as a taken-for-granted problem in contemporary societies. In this sense, sociologists and other social scientists seek to deconstruct the very idea of an obesity pandemic.

Goffman's (1963) often cited work on stigma also provides a useful way of understanding the relationship between fatness and social status (for a discussion of stigma also see Chapter 1). Stigma refers to an attribute that is deeply discrediting (Goffman, 1963), disqualifying a person from full participation in society, and setting him or her aside as deviant, rather than 'normal'. Goffman makes the distinction between individual physical attributes that are discreditable and those which are discrediting. Discreditable attributes are those which can usually be easily hidden from others, for example, diabetes or HIV. Discrediting attributes cannot be hidden from others and are immediately stigmatizing for the individual concerned. Obesity and overweight are good examples of a discrediting attribute. Goffman suggests that the attribution of responsibility for stigma is important in that individuals are more likely to be stigmatized if they are seen as responsible for their discrediting attribute. Overweight and obese people are often seen as responsible for their weight – they may be perceived as greedy, lazy and lacking in willpower. For obese people, fatness can become what Goffman terms their 'master status' – the quality or characteristic which defines the individual above all others. As discussed in Chapter 1, stigma can also be experienced as either 'felt' or 'enacted'; felt stigma referring to the direct consequences of a discrediting attribute and enacted stigma to the expectation of negative consequences. Both of these may be relevant to people's experiences of defining themselves, or being defined as 'fat', 'obese' or 'overweight'. For example, a qualitative Scottish study of 36 obese, overweight and 'normal' weight young people

(Wills et al., 2006) found that participants referred to being 'fat', both as a description of body size or shape and as a term of abuse. Approximately half of the participants in this study who were obese or overweight reported being bullied simply because of their weight. Similarly, in an in-depth qualitative study of 9 obese women living in New Zealand, Carryer (2001) describes women's experiences of chronic reduction – or yo-yo – dieting, obsessions with food, and feelings of shame and stigma. She describes the impact of obesity on women's access to health and health care. For example, one respondent in this study said:

> Once going into A & E [emergency room] with suspected appendicitis, I was feeling really miserable. They left me there and then poked and prodded around of course and this doctor came in and he said of course you are overweight, and I thought well that was a brilliant deduction, I said 'so it can't possibly be appendicitis then, you know it's just fat?' (Carryer, 2001, p. 95)

Goffman (1963) also refers to the concept of 'courtesy stigma', where the stigma associated with one individual is also felt or enacted by close friends and family. For example, in Monaghan's (2007a, b) study of men, masculinities and weight, one man reported that his children were bullied on account of his weight.

Sontag's (1979, 1989) work on illness and metaphor (see Chapter 1) can also offer a useful insight into understanding the significance of obesity and overweight within contemporary societies. Focusing specifically on cancer and HIV Sontag explores how certain illnesses (and in particular those which are poorly understood) come to be known as much more than just an illness or long-term condition. For example, for many years the word 'cancer' has been synonymous with death – with this metaphor having had far-reaching consequences for the prevention and treatment of many cancers. The concept of illness and metaphor can also usefully be applied to obesity and overweight in that obesity has become widely accepted as a metaphor for individual sloth, greed and abundance. For example, writing in the Guardian about children and obesity, Parry (2005, online) argues, 'To be overweight is said to be the product of a breakdown in family values and of slothful kids.' Of course, such moralizing is not new. Indeed, there is a long cultural history of the association between fatness and morality and the responsibility of individuals and families – especially mothers – for food and health (Gard and Wright, 2005). Indeed, these metaphors are found everywhere. For example, the House of Commons Health Committee Report on obesity stated:

> It is certain that obesity develops only when there is a sustained imbalance between the amount of energy consumed by a person and the amount used up in everyday life. But which side of this energy balance equation has been most altered in recent decades to produce such rapid weight gain? Should obesity be blamed on gluttony, sloth, or both? (House of Commons, 2004)

Sontag's insight into the use of metaphor in relation to illness continues to be influential in social science understandings of long term conditions.

Lay understandings of obesity and overweight owe as much to biomedical and epidemiological approaches as to 'common sense' views such as those derived from the mass media. Of course, the mass media derive its (mis)understandings from biomedical and epidemiological viewpoints and, when depicting obesity, often adopts the metaphor of war. For example, one headline in the Guardian reads: 'Hormone raises hope of victory in war on obesity' (Jha, 2005, online) and another in the Observer reads: 'US sugar barons "block global war on obesity"' (Revill and Harris, 2004, online). The media also continue to perpetuate the notion of obesity as a social and moral problem, rather than just a biomedical one. The proliferation of television programmes such as *The Biggest Loser* (NBC, 2007) *Fat Families* (ITV1, 2005) or *Honey We're Killing the Kids* (BBC3, 2005) pay testimony to this and, specifically, to the view that the obesity epidemic is caused by individual and familial gluttony and sloth, for example:

> Do you have young children? Take a look at them. Now, can you imagine being introduced to them ... when they're grown up? What if the future you'd imagined for them hasn't quite gone to plan? How would you react if you discovered that, as adults, your children have under-achieved, have serious health problems and have a much lower than average life expectancy? And, as their parents,

it's all **your** fault! (BBC3, *Honey We're Killing the Kids,* 2005, original emphasis)

Of course, media representations of obesity should be contextualized within wider discourses on food, body image and weight. Whilst the media continues to perpetuate the notion that obesity is a social and moral problem, as well as a medical one, increasing alarm is also being raised over the phenomenon of celebrity slimness and the 'size 0'. For example, Spencer, writing in *The Observer* argues:

> ... Lindsay Lohan, Mischa Barton, Nicole Richie, Kate Bosworth, Amy Winehouse – women relatively new on the celebrity radar who skitter across the pages of magazines, coat hangers furnished with tennis-ball boobs and expensive shoes, not a shred of fat to share among them. You might not give a tossed salad how much these bony birds weigh. You might even agree with Kate Hudson (who recently won a libel action against the UK National Enquirer magazine for implying she had an eating disorder) that it is none of our business. But it is. It matters because hyper-thin has somehow become today's celebrity standard and, as a result – almost without us noticing – the goalposts have moved for us all. (Spencer, 2006, online)

Drawing on scientific knowledge in their reporting of obesity, media representations are usually warning of a catastrophic global obesity epidemic in which everyone, everywhere, is at risk (Gard and Wright, 2005). Writing specifically about the role of the media and its contribution to the construction of an obesity epidemic in the United States, Boero (2007) suggests that, unlike the construction of traditional epidemics (which are characterized by contagion and mass death), those at risk of becoming obese are as central to the obesity epidemic as those who actually are obese or overweight. Boero argues:

> ... we all have to eat, and therefore, we are all 'at risk' and must be vigilant. This fear of fat is perpetuated by the idea that anyone can become fat at any time and with little effort, that becoming fat is both outside of one's normal control yet also eminently within it ... only those who obsess and display behaviours that are often negatively associated with eating disorders and food compulsions have even the slightest chance at avoiding becoming fat or maintaining even 'moderate' weight loss. (Boero, 2007, p. 47)

Mass media representations of obesity are important. They can influence the way that lay people (and others) understand and experience obesity, though they never reflect the totality of these experiences. As discussed in the next section, the nursing profession can – and should – play a role in mediating the messages perpetuated by the media.

Treating and preventing obesity: Health care and the role of nurses

In spite of the high profile of obesity and overweight within government policy, health agencies, health care, the media and amongst lay people, reports indicate that obese patients are not able to access the weight management services they need from Primary Care Trusts (PCTs) (*Nursing Standard*, 2005). In fact, many PCTs do not have established weight management clinics, and those that do are understandably overstretched with very long waiting lists for those lucky enough to be placed on them. Writing in the Nursing Standard (2007), Anne Diamond – broadcaster and health campaigner – who draws on her personal experiences of managing obesity, asks:

> If you are overweight and want to do something about it, where do you go? The sensible answer might seem to be your GP practice. Unfortunately, you are likely to be disappointed and humiliated. This is because your GP will simply push a diet sheet towards you and utter the mantra: 'Just eat less and exercise more.' We are in the grip of an epidemic...yet health professionals are treating a worsening crisis with a post-war mentality and a ration book. (Diamond, 2007, p. 26)

Most health professionals, and others, agree that something needs to be done about the obesity pandemic and in spite of government commitment to the prevention of obesity, funds have not been successfully ring-fenced for that purpose. The BBC journalist, Paul Barltrop (BBC online, 2006) argues that whilst the plans for health trainers and extra school nurses, dieticians and health psychologists sound good, when trusts are operating over-budget, extra funds are easily diverted. This has led many commentators to argue that governments need to intervene more directly in improving health and well-being, even if that means impinging on personal choice and freedom. For example, in an editorial published in the *British Journal of Community Nursing*, Pollard (2004) argues that 'we need a hand from nanny' and states: '...personal choice has failed the population, and will lead to a significant health and financial burden. In such a case, government intervention has become not only desirable, but absolutely necessary' (Pollard, 2004, p. 236).

Whilst there is no agreement on this position, it remains true that nurses (and other health professionals) can play a key role in the treatment of people who are obese and overweight and in the prevention of obesity. However, given the insights offered by sociological perspectives on obesity and overweight it is, perhaps, wise to be cautious before jumping on the bandwagon that has become the obesity pandemic.

McHugh (2006) argues that the general public has received conflicting messages regarding obesity and overweight over the last few years. The scientific debate on obesity continues to evolve but McHugh highlights how the media and interest groups (such as the food industry) can spin the information in ways that are either unhelpful and confusing, or downright dishonest. He suggests that nurses should play a greater role in mediating this health information by working collaboratively with others to ensure that research is interpreted honestly and appropriately and that clear messages are given to the general public. He argues that many nurses are in a unique position to provide fundamental public health information on obesity but that to do so, nurses must be aware of the way in which diverse interest groups can misinterpret information, thus helping patients and clients to disentangle the messages they receive. Chang et al. (2004) also examine the role of nurses and go further to suggest that, in order to promote public health, nurses should play a more active role in the politics of obesity and overweight. However, writing specifically about the role of the specialist nurse, Banning (2005) suggests that to enable nurses to engage in these activities, the nursing profession needs to rise to the challenge of obesity and must prepare nurses for a specialist role in obesity management.

There have been several studies carried out to explore nurses' attitudes to overweight and obese patients and the impact of these on service quality and outcomes for obese people. For example, in a qualitative study carried out in the United Kingdom, Wright (1998) suggests that nurses can feel uneasy about assessing weight or discussing weight with patients. A study carried out in Canada and the United States (Petrich, 2000) reports that nurses often feel repulsion for obese patients, seeing them as lazy and lacking in self-control. Female patients, in particular, were often judged more harshly than men for being obese or overweight. Mercer and Tessier (2001), in another qualitative study carried out in the United Kingdom, note that nurses often have little enthusiasm for working with obese patients, citing a lack of motivation on the part of patients as the main cause of this. Most other studies show similar results. In a review of the quantitative and qualitative literature on nurses' attitudes to obese patients, Brown (2006) argues that given the negative attitudes of society towards obesity, it is not surprising that nurses have negative attitudes towards obese patients. He argues that these attitudes are important because of their negative implications for the quality of healthcare and because they may prevent individuals from accessing services.

Conclusion

Arguably, although the treatment and prevention of obesity and overweight should be a significant priority within healthcare, the issue remains a low priority for many nurses, doctors and other health care professionals. A sociological perspective on obesity highlights the importance of the social in understanding not only the experiences of those who are obese or overweight, but the way in which the social helps shape the construction of a long-term condition.

There is clearly some scope for reflection on personal beliefs on obesity and on behaviour towards patients or clients (and colleagues) who are obese and overweight. There is also some room for improvement in the provision of appropriate and timely services and interventions. There is much to be achieved within the health care services, and particularly by nurses, to ensure that people who are obese or overweight receive appropriate treatment and, more widely, to ensure that obesity can be prevented in the future. As Munro argues:

> This is a time for nurses to quietly reflect on their own attitudes and beliefs about obesity and to join forces and campaign together for the equal and fair treatment of obese patients in the face of political pressure to achieve equity, user involvement and social inclusion for this vulnerable group. (Munro, 2006, p. 748)

References

Banning M., 'The management of obesity: the role of the specialist nurse', *British Journal of Nursing*, 14: 3 (2005) 139–144.

Barltrop P., 'The vanishing £800,000', *The Politics Show West*, BBC News (online, 2006) http://news.bbc.co.uk/1/hi/programmes/politics_show/6129180.stm (last accessed 19 September 2007).

BBC3, 'Honey We're Killing the Kids' (2005) http://www.bbc.co.uk/bbcthree/tv/killing_the_kids.shtml (last accessed 9 April 2006).

Boero N., 'All the news that's fat to print: The American "obesity epidemic" and the media', *Qualitative Sociology*, 30 (2007) 41–60.

Bordo S., *Unbearable Weight: Feminism, Western Culture and the Body* (London: University of California Press, 1995).

British Medical Association (BMA) *Preventing Childhood Obesity* (London: BMA, 2005).

Brown I., 'Nurses' attitudes towards adult patients who are obese: literature review', *Journal of Advanced Nursing*, 53: 3 (2006) 221–232.

Brownell K.D., 'The chronicling of obesity: growing awareness of its social, economic, and political contexts', *Journal of Health Politics, Policy and Law*, 30: 5 (2005) 955–964.

Carr D., and M.A. Friedman, 'Is obesity stigmatizing? Body weight, perceived discrimination, and psychological well-being in the United States', *Journal of Health and Social Behavior*, 46: 3 (2005) 244–259.

Carryer J., 'Embodied largeness: a significant women's health issue', *Nursing Inquiry*, 8: 2 (2001) 90–97.

Chang Y-M, Y-M Liou, S-J Sheu and M-Y Chen, 'Unbearable weight: young adult women's experiences of being overweight', *Journal of Nursing Research*, 12: 2 (2004) 153–159.

Chernin K., *Womansize: the Tyranny of Slenderness* (London: The Women's Press, 1981).

Conway R., and A. Rene 'Obesity as a disease: no lightweight matter', *Obesity Reviews*, 5 (2004) 145–151.

Cooper C., 'Can a fat woman call herself disabled?', *Disability & Society*, 12: 1 (1997) 31–41.

Davidson M., and K.A. Knafl, 'Dimensional analysis of the concept of obesity', *Journal of Advanced Nursing*, 54: 3 (2006) 342–350.

Department of Health (DH), *Choosing Health: Making Healthy Choices Easier* (London: The Stationery Office, 2004).

Deurenberg P., and M. Deurenberg-Yap, 'Differences in body composition assumptions across ethnic groups: practical consequences', *Current Opinion in Clinical Nutrition and Metabolic Care*, 4 (2001) 377–383.

Deurenberg P., M. Deurenberg-Yap and S. Guricci, 'Asians are different from Caucasians and from each other in their body mass index/body fat per cent relationship', *Obesity Reviews*, 3 (2002) 141–146.

Diamond A., 'Why obesity is the new smoking', *Nursing Standard*, 21: 26 (2007) 26–27.

Doll H.A., S.E.K. Peterson and S.L. Stewart-Brown, 'Obesity and physical and emotional well-being: associations between body mass index, chronic illness and the physical and mental components of the SF-36 questionnaire', *Obesity Research*, 8: 2 (2000) 160–170.

Gard M., and J. Wright, *The Obesity Epidemic: Science, Morality and Ideology* (London: Routledge, 2005).

Goffman E., *Stigma: Notes on the Study of a Spoiled Identity* (London: Penguin Books, 1963).

M. Heo M., A. Pietrobelli, K.R. Fontaine, J.A. Sirey and M.S. Faith, 'Depressive mood and obesity in US adults: comparison and moderation by sex, age and race', *International Journal of Obesity*, 30: 3 (2006) 513–519.

House of Commons Health Committee, *Obesity: Third Report of Session 2003–4* (London: The Stationery Office, 2004).

Hunt K., 'A "cure for all ills?" constructions of the menopause and the chequered fortunes of hormone replacement therapy', in S. Wilkinson and C. Kitzinger (eds), *Women and Health: Feminist Perspectives.* (London: Taylor & Francis, 1994).

Jha A., 'Hormone raises hope of victory in war on obesity', *Guardian* (2005) November 11.

Lee C., *Women's Health: Psychological and Social Perspectives* (London: Sage, 1998).

McHugh M.D., 'Fit or fat? A review of the debate on deaths attributable to obesity', *Public Health Nursing*, 23: 3 (2006) 264–270.

Mercer S., and S. Tessier, 'A qualitative study of general practitioners' and practice nurses' attitudes to obesity management in primary care', *Health Bulletin*, 59 (2001) 248–253.

Monaghan L.F., 'Body mass index, masculinities and moral worth: men's critical understandings of "appropriate" weight-for-height', *Sociology of Health & Illness*, 29: 4 (2007a) 584–609.

Monaghan L.F., 'McDonaldizing men's bodies? slimming, associated (ir)rationalities and resistances', *Body & Society*, 13: 2 (2007b) 67–93.

Munro J., 'It's time for nurses to get behind obese patients', *British Journal of Nursing*, 15: 14 (2006) 748.

Neovius M., Y. Linné, B. Barkeling and S. Rössner, 'Discrepancies between classification systems of childhood obesity', *Obesity Reviews*, 5 (2004) 105–114.

Nursing Standard, 'Half of trusts lack obesity clinics', 19: 23 (2005) 8.

Orbach S., *Fat is a Feminist Issue* (London: Arrow Books, 1988).

Parry V., 'Fat versus fiction', *The Guardian*, Thursday 16 June (2005) http://www.guardian.co.uk/life/lastword/story/0,,1506961,00. html (last accessed 9 April 2006).

Petrich B., 'Medical and nursing students' perceptions of obesity', *Journal of Addictions Nursing*, 14 (2000) 744–754.

Pollard T., 'Tackling obesity: we need a hand from nanny', *British Journal of Community Nursing*, 9: 6 (2004) 236.

Revill J., and P. Harris, 'US sugar barons "block global war on obesity"', *Observer* (2004) Sunday January 18.

Sjoberg R.L., K.W. Nilsson and J. Leppert, 'Obesity, shame, and depression in school-aged children: a population-based study', *Pediatrics*, 116: 3 (2005) 389–392.

Sontag S., *Illness and Metaphor* (London: Allen Lane, 1979).

Sontag S., *AIDS and its Metaphors* (London: Penguin, 1989).

Spencer M., 'The shape we're in', *The Observer*, online (2006) Sunday 6 Augusthttp://observer.guardian.co.uk/woman/story/ 0,,1835485,00.html (last accessed 10 October 2007).

Templeton S.K., 'Nurses fight weight test for children', *The Sunday Times*, July 17 (2005) 5.

Wardle J., and L. Cooke, 'The impact of obesity on psychological well-being', *Best Practice & Research Clinical Endocrinology & Metabolism*, 19: 3 (2005) 421–440.

Wills W., K. Backett-Milburn, S. Gregory and J. Lawton, ' "Young teenagers" perceptions of their own and others' bodies: a qualitative study of obese, overweight and "normal" weight young people in Scotland', *Social Science & Medicine*, 62 (2006) 396–406.

World Health Organisation (WHO), *Diet, Nutrition and the Prevention of Chronic Diseases: Report of a Joint WHO/FAO Expert Consultation* (Geneva: WHO, 2003).

World Health Organisation (WHO), *Obesity: Preventing and Managing the Global Epidemic*, WHO Technical Report Series 894 (Geneva: WHO, 2000).

Wright J., 'Female nurses' perceptions of acceptable female body size: an exploratory study', *Journal of Clinical Nursing*, 7 (1998) 307–315.

Zola I.K., 'Pathways to the doctor – from person to patient', *Social Science & Medicine*, 7 (1973) 766–789.

12

Heartsink patients and intractable conditions

Elaine Denny

A couple of days before my second operation he calls me a hypochondriac. I mean I used to hate going to see him. As soon as I opened the door he would say 'Oh you again'.

(Denny, 2004a, p. 42)

This quotation epitomizes the feelings of people who have what are known by the medical profession as 'heartsink' conditions, or are viewed as 'heartsink' patients. They have an illness or condition that is long term, is causing them pain and/or other distressing symptoms, for which either no cause has yet been found or no treatment has been successful to date. Heartsink describes the feeling of the doctor or other health professional on seeing these patients walk through the door yet again, when s/he has nothing new to offer them in order to improve their symptoms. Yet for the patient, despite the fact that previous treatments have not been successful they frequently perceive that they have no other option but to return to the health professionals who are the gatekeepers to all other health services.

The term heartsink was coined by O'Dowd in the late 1980s to describe those patients who 'evoke an overwhelming mixture of exasperation, defeat and sometimes plain dislike that causes the heart to sink when they consult.' (O'Dowd, 1988, p. 528). A heartsink patient is always identified and defined by the doctor, and it is the doctor's experience of an individual that induces the label.

Characteristics of what constitutes heartsink have been identified as including psychosomatic illness, lower social class, being female, having thick clinical records, and making frequent use of the health services. Butler and Evans (1999) also point to heartsink behaviour as persistent visits, unresolved clinical symptoms and difficulties in defining clinical problems. However, O'Dowd states that heartsink patients are in fact a disparate group, who often have serious medical problems, and whose only common feature is the distress they cause to their doctor. Illingworth (1988) suggests that it is the doctor's impatience, intolerance, fatigue or pressure of work that leads to irritation with patients. So ascribing a label has the effect of locating the problem with the patient, whereas it may well lie with the medical professional, or with the health care system.

Taking a more sociological approach involves looking beyond the individual players, and focusing on structural issues around the types of medical problems likely to lead to pejorative labels. The factors that link the conditions are first, the absence of consensual biomedical facts. Rather they are characterized by diverse kinds of knowledge (both lay and professional), experience and power relations (Brown, 1995), and ideas about how to manage them. Second, they are frequently not of interest medically speaking, although whether this is cause or effect is difficult to assess; is knowledge not produced because these illnesses are not of interest medically, or are they not of interest because there is not a research base or successful treatment for them? Bury (1991), in his review of research on chronic illness, pointed to a number of factors that could impact on the individual's attempt to maintain personal integrity and reduce the threat to social status in the face of radically altered circumstances. One such factor is a disease that is neither of great medical interest or widely publicly recognized. Finally, the presenting symptoms are not characteristic of a particular disease, and may be commonly experienced. Again Bury (1991, p. 456) notes that some conditions 'may produce symptoms, which because of their widespread occurrence in milder forms, among the normal population, make legitimation extremely difficult.' In Western biomedicine legitimation is generally via diagnosis by a health professional, usually a doctor. One of the initial problems encountered by people suffering from physical symptoms of some kind is in receiving a diagnosis, and so a consideration of diagnosis, of categorizing those symptoms and legitimizing the sufferer by giving them a name, is an important starting point.

Brown (1995) states that diagnosis is integral to the theory and practice of modern Western medicine. Waitzskin (1989) also points to the strong drive to reach a diagnosis, the view among doctors instilled from medical training that it is one of the most important medical skills. Interruption or redirection of the patient by the professional is often directed at emphasizing the parts of the patient's story that are consistent with previously defined diagnostic categories with which the professional is familiar, and playing down other parts. Waitzkin describes diagnostic reasoning as 'both limited and exclusionary' (1989, p. 230) in that it excludes a large part of the patient's experience that is important to them, but not considered relevant to the medical diagnosis. The medical plan that follows diagnosis also marginalizes social context, treatment options frequently being limited to technical ones such as medication or surgery, occasionally prevention or lifestyle change. This lack of attention to the patient experience or social context is not the inadequacy of medical training as much as a reflection of what medicine is in Western society; that is, a scientific and technical discipline. Williams (2003) comments on the uncertainty surrounding chronic illness: uncertainty over diagnosis, over the course of the disease, and over the future as a key feature of the experience of living with chronic illness. This is particularly true of the early stages when symptoms may be the result of a number of pathological conditions, or some variation of normal experience.

Many sociologists (e.g., Atkinson, 1977; Fox, 2000) have pointed to the guided discovery process by which the presenting complaints and symptoms become interpreted into an 'organised illness' (Brown, 1995, p. 39). Similarly Balint in his seminal work of 1957 talked of unorganized illness being organized by the doctor. This is often uncontested, but it is in conflictual illnesses that issues of power and control over legitimation of illness are brought into sharp relief.

Of relevance here is the medicalization of facets of normal life, what Illich (1976) has termed social *iatrogenesis*, where processes are redefined as medical problems and labelled as such. This is not however always a case of medical expansionism or social control as people who experience certain conditions may well seek a diagnosis as a way of legitimating that experience. This may be in order to excuse themselves from normal roles (see Chapter 1 for a discussion of the sick role) but it may also be necessary to legitimate their symptoms to themselves or to others in order to maintain self esteem.

In some illnesses, definitions are contested in that although they are generally accepted there is no widely applied medical definition, in other words the collection of symptoms is accepted as legitimate, but there is no agreed diagnosis by which to 'organise' them. An example here is what has come to be known as Gulf War Syndrome. The symptoms experienced by Veterans are accepted as genuine, but the organization of those symptoms as a specific syndrome is not universally accepted by the medical profession, neither is the Gulf War universally accepted as aetiology.

A model of the stages of social construction of disease has been developed by Brown (1995). First disease must be identified and diagnosed as such; the social discovery of disease. Medical science may encourage or resist discovery. Social policy also plays a part in the identification of disease by the awarding of research grants and by directing funding into certain priority areas. Once a disease has been discovered people experience it quite differently and the experience of illness constitutes the second stage. Singular medical typologies are often at variance with sociological ones that acknowledge individual experience and also the differences in perception that arise from societal structures such as social class, gender, ethnicity and age. The lay and professional construction of disease is not however totally separate as understandings of health and illness are to a large degree informed by the dominant biomedical model, particularly in non-conflictual disease, such as diabetes, so patient and professional ideas are influenced by the same cultural values.

The third stage, treatment, is a logical sequel to diagnosis and experience, and what are deemed appropriate ways to treat illness are socially constructed. Whether a person seeks medical care, alternative therapy, self or lay care is dependent on many factors, including social economic circumstances, health beliefs and interpretation of presenting symptoms. Within organized health systems what treatment a person receives maybe the result of macro policy decisions, personal preferences of individual health professionals, or influenced by outside forces such as the pharmaceutical industry. When to withdraw treatment is also largely an ad hoc decision, based on macro and micro policy decisions. The final stage of the process is outcome, which raises questions about how 'success' of treatment is measured. Organizational factors often determine belief in success, for example cancer services have traditionally been judged on five year survival rates. The criteria for medical outcomes are frequently measurable results, whereas patients and their families may have different criteria, which may be harder to define and quantify. With heartsink conditions or patients there are tensions between lay and professional perspectives on what constitutes successful treatment, and who defines it.

From the discussion above three themes can be identified that are relevant to a discussion of the concepts of heartsink patients and intractable conditions, and that prove problematic for the experience of chronic illness. They are problems surrounding diagnosis and treatment, conditions that are not of interest to the medical profession, and conditions that are characterized by symptoms that are widespread in milder form in the general population. These three themes will be illuminated in the following sections by a discussion of three long-term conditions (chronic back pain, endometriosis, and Irritable Bowel Syndrome [IBS]) where the illness experience is often negative.

Chronic back pain

Low back pain is a common problem suffered by the most of the adult population at some time in their lives. Although for most the experience is short lived, some people suffer recurrent bouts, and for others the condition becomes chronic and they suffer almost constant pain. Yet the cause is often elusive in that there is not always any obvious damage to the spine, and the pain is frequently not associated with a serious illness. Back pain provides a useful illustration of the problems faced in getting a diagnosis for people with symptoms that are widespread in the population.

Glenton (2003) conducted in-depth interviews and obtained data from an online discussion group for back pain sufferers. The original focus of the research was to discover information needs of people with back pain, but it soon became apparent that of major importance to participants was having their pain accepted as real, and not being thought of as malingerers or hypochondriacs. As has been discussed in Chapter 1 the sick role has been criticized for its inapplicability for chronic illness. Yet though accepting that the rights and obligations are not appropriate for chronic illness, Glenton argues that the sick role concept does reflect the social obligations and expectations present in the minds of health professionals, colleagues, family, and the back pain sufferers themselves. In other words, the biomedical model is so dominant that the legitimation of pain is bound up with the ability to demonstrate appropriate clinical and social characteristics.

For example, one participant's comment reflects very well the sick role obligation to want to get well: 'When you're not getting any further, you're just on sick leave, you're not getting any treatment, nothings happening, right. "Well how ill are you?" I notice from people around me: "isn't anything happening? Aren't you going to get treatment? What's happening? Are you just going to lie there?" ' (Glenton, 2003, p. 2247).

Glenton concludes that the greatest threat to back pain sufferers' social status is the suspicion that the pain does not really exist, and that the expectations of the sick role lead people with low back pain to fit into the system by striving to live up to them.

One way of achieving legitimation is to have a positive test or some visible 'proof' of disease. Rhodes et al. (2002) explored the motivation of people with low back pain to keep returning for medical care when conventional treatment offers them little relief from pain. They found that issues of testing, legitimation and visibility were tightly linked in the interviews, and argue that 'the concern with the visual representation of illness expressed ... has roots in biomedical and popular attitudes that privilege this form of representation.' (Rhodes et al., 2000, p. 37). This anatomical understanding of the body is premised on two assumptions – that the inside of the body corresponds to visual images of it, and that there are objective norms from which variations in individual bodies can be measured. The role of the doctor here is to look at the visual images and to discover deviations from the assumed normal spine.

Naturally then, the participants in the study of Rhodes et al., felt that seeing a cause made their pain real and justified their persistence, as the following quote demonstrates: 'I felt relieved. I felt like, well, here's proof. It's not just me going crazy or complaining. It's black and white and anybody can see it.' (Rhodes et al., 2000, p. 38).

Paradoxically those participants in the study of Rhodes et al., who did not have their pain explained by visual test results criticized the doctor's reliance on testing, and felt delegitimized in the absence of visual proof. The authors conclude that diagnostic testing is a two-edged sword. It often fails to provide a meaningful explanation for pain and the patient is left with a sense of deficiency and shame.

Miller and Timson (2004), in their study on partners of people with low back pain, found that they had little faith in the knowledge of the professionals who were encountered. The partners' opinion was that they did not behave like 'experts'. Their expectation of experts was that they should act proactively and give explanations for the condition. In the absence of this the impression was that nothing was being done for their partner. There was also the view expressed that the medical profession made value laden judgements based on the diagnosis and labelled back pain sufferers as shirking social or economic duties. As one participant commented

> I honestly believe that you're tarred with the same brush and that you're trying to rake the system. ... I have to watch the pain every day where you can go and see a doctor for one day, who may be having a bad day, and you're looked upon as if you're just a fraud. (Miller and Timson, 2004, p. 39–40)

In a secondary analysis of their own data designed to elicit how General Practitioners (GPs) conceptualize chronic illness in the consultation, May et al. (2004) demonstrated an incongruence between the patient's account of an organic pathology, and the doctor's account which used a psycho-social model to explain symptoms. So legitimacy of the symptoms and motivation for the patient presenting them extend to disagreement about the pathological processes involved, but in this case the doctor's attempt to use a non-medical model is overwhelmed by the strength of the biomedical model. One GP stated 'You can't get them to accept this [lack of organic pathology] (...) If you really upset them, they're not going to trust you again.' (May et al., 2004, p. 146 original parentheses). As the patient's symptoms and subjective experience were not adequately explained by tests that yielded little, GPs defined them as psychogenic or social in origin, which made action to relieve them problematic. Another reading of the data provided here is that the GPs are also heavily reliant on the biomedical model. This is demonstrated by the way in which lack of diagnostic 'proof' of disease was not interpreted as a limitation in the mechanisms for testing, but as the patient having a non-medical problem.

The problem for the GP in the absence of any action to 'cure' the symptoms is one of containment, which the patient may construe as a failure of the medical system. For the GP, who could not provide effective therapy, nor reach agreement with the patient on how to understand their problem, the result was frustration. The reanalysis of this research was contrasted in the study with research on menorrhagia and depression, both conditions where there was relative certainty in the efficacy of the biomedical model in diagnosis of and response to symptoms, even though for both conditions effectiveness of treatments was equivocal.

This literature demonstrates that back pain provides a useful illustration of the themes of the chapter in that it constitutes a condition where diagnosis is difficult, and frequently the available diagnostic procedures produce no satisfactory outcome for the patient. The absence of a diagnosis resulted in people lacking legitimacy, and particularly with a symptom that is widespread among the population generally, sufferers felt the need to have some proof or professional acceptance to distinguish their pain.

Endometriosis

Endometriosis is a chronic condition in which endometrial tissue is present outside of the uterus, usually but not always in the abdominal cavity. The cyclical hormonal influence on these endometrial deposits causes bleeding into places where it cannot escape, leading to the typical symptom of severe pelvic pain. As this is frequently experienced during menstruation symptoms are regarded as widespread and normal and therefore, in common with back pain, are of little interest to the medical profession.

However, for symptomatic women the pain can be overwhelming. Graphic descriptions of the pain feature in most research, such as 'like a knife' and 'nails clawing inside your stomach' (Denny, 2004b, p. 644); 'gnawing' and 'like sitting on a knitting needle' (Huntington and Gilmour, 2005, p. 1128). Novelist Hilary Mantle describes her experience of endometrial pain thus:

> At 18, I went on the pill. My period pains eased, but soon nausea, vomiting, fatigue and aching legs took me to the doctor. These symptoms lasted through the month, and no one added them up. I was offered tranquillisers and anti-depressants, and the opportunity of life as a psychiatric patient, which in the end I found the strength to decline.
>
> Throughout my 20s I sought a diagnosis for increasing debility. Doctors read my notes and wrote me off. When I left off the pill, menstruation became agony; every part of my body seemed to hurt. When I was 27 – a skinny, grey faced scrap, bleeding continuously and hardly able to stand up – my disease was named. (Mantle, 2004)

Lemaire (2004) found in her study of the symptoms of endometriosis that women experienced multiple symptoms, and varying levels of distress, including symptoms not normally associated with endometriosis, and other literature reports that living with endometriosis has a profound impact on women. Their social and work relationships, their sexuality, and indeed their ability to function are all affected by it (Denny, 2004b; Jones et al., 2004).

In common with people who suffer back pain, women with endometriosis experience a delay in diagnosis. Hadfield et al. (1996) reported that in the United Kingdom the mean length of time between onset of pain and laparoscopic diagnosis is 7.96 years and in the US ten years, a longer period than for other chronic diseases, such as rheumatoid arthritis. Delay in diagnosis is also reported by other research on endometriosis.

Jones et al. (2004) attribute it in part to the fact that many women are initially misdiagnosed, in particular with IBS. Ballard et al. (2006) categorized diagnostic delays as occurring at a patient level and at a medical level. Cox et al. (2003) report women 'doctor shopping' to find someone who will take their symptoms seriously, and not dismiss their pain as something they have to put up with.

Much research reports that women describe their GP as either disinterested in as possessing a very poor knowledge of endometriosis, and a number also make this claim regarding gynaecologists. One woman in Denny and Mann (2008, p. 113) reported her GP as saying 'I don't know this condition at all'. So they feel that their symptoms are not treated seriously, and often report feeling fobbed off or dismissed in encounters with the medical profession. Women frequently use the terms 'battle' or 'struggle' to describe their attempts to be taken seriously. The consequence of this for many women is the delay in diagnosis of their symptoms as endometriosis, as discussed above.

A compounding issue for women with endometriosis is the association with menstruation. Women report that their symptoms are normalized and treated as if they were the result of the physiological process of menstruation, rather than something pathological, such as the woman who said 'I went to the doctor's and he said "Women do suffer with painful periods, it's one of those things."' (Denny 2004a, p. 40). In medical and lay circles menstrual pain is treated as normal, just part of being a woman and women who cannot manage it are made to feel that they are inadequate and overreacting at best, and neurotic and depressed at worst. Ballard et al. (2006) also found that family doctors normalized the pain of endometriosis, but stated that women too had difficulty in distinguishing between 'normal' and 'abnormal' menstrual experience.

In Bendelow's (1993) research on pain and gender the view was expressed by both men and women in the interview sample that biology and their reproductive role made women 'naturally' more able to endure pain, both physical and emotional, which in turn led to the expectation that they could put up with more pain than men, and that perhaps their pain would not have to be taken as seriously. For women with endometriosis this compounds the notion that period pain is a normal part of the menstrual cycle, and therefore something that has to be lived with. So notions of how women experience pain, coupled with ideas of coping with menstrual pain both add to the difficulty for women with endometriosis in having their illness legitimized.

Although a detailed history can be highly indicative of endometriosis, the 'gold standard' diagnosis is by laparoscopy, when lesions can be visualized and biopsies taken. Seeing the endometriotic lesions on video or photographs added to patients' sense of credibility, and this is consistent with Rhodes et al. (2002) above. However, this visualization does not provide legitimation in the straightforward way of Rhodes' et al., study on back pain. A feature of endometriosis is that the severity of symptoms of endometriosis does not necessarily correlate with the extent of disease, and yet biomedical categorization is by a linear progression from minimal to severe (or stage 1 to 4). A woman who is diagnosed as having 'mild' disease according to diagnostic categorization may experience severe pain, while another who has extensive disease may be asymptomatic, and is only diagnosed opportunistically, for example at the time of laparoscopic sterilization or during investigations for infertility. One participant in Denny and Mann (2008, p. 113) who was experiencing severe pain said of her GP, 'He obviously had no idea how this disease can affect you at all. He told me "you've only got spots of [endometriosis], lots of women have that and they get on with their life" '.

When women do finally get a diagnosis, the initial reaction is usually one of relief, followed by a sense of vindication. They have an explanation of what is happening to them, and are not mad or hypochondriac, which are labels a number of women have ascribed to them. This vindication is in turn often followed by anger at the number of years they had spent in pain, and the effect on their lives and relationships that may have been avoided with earlier treatment: 'When they gave me my endo diagnosis I was fuming that I hadn't been believed and that I hadn't been taken seriously ... I was actually convinced by a doctor that I was psychosomatic and a bit of a hypochondriac' (Denny, 2004a, p. 41).

This section has shown how many women with endometriosis find that the medical profession is largely disinterested in symptoms that they consider a normal part of the physiological process of menstruation, and also the gendered nature of the construction of pain. This, in turn, leads to a delay in diagnosis. Legitimation of symptoms, an acceptance that they are not normal, is needed for women to be believed and taken seriously. Dysmenorrhoea is experienced by many women, and not only doctors but also the woman herself and those around her may display scepticism to the symptoms of endometriosis.

Irritable bowel syndrome (IBS)

Irritable Bowel syndrome is a painful condition characterized by diarrhoea, constipation, cramping abdominal pain and bloating. In common with the conditions discussed above, it is painful and distressing, but not life threatening. Moreover there is no specific diagnostic test or observable pathology and so IBS is often diagnosed following negative tests for other diseases, or in the absence of any firm explanation for symptoms. Diagnosis is often made using checklists, such as the Manning criteria or the ROME criteria (Talley, Boyce and Jones, 1997), which are codifications of symptoms. However, in a review of the literature Whitehead, et al. (2002) report that the criteria for a diagnosis of IBS in studies varies from self report by questionnaire to unspecified symptom criteria.

IBS would appear to have much in common with low back pain and endometriosis, in that it that it is a disease of little interest to the medical profession and manifests with symptomatology that is common in the wider population. Sufferers often experience a delay in diagnosis, and they frequently find themselves disbelieved and their symptoms trivialised. Moreover Talley et al. (1997) suggest that management of IBS remains unsatisfactory because the cause is obscure. Despite these tensions IBS has not been the focus of sociological enquiry in the same way as low back pain and endometriosis. The dominant approach to researching IBS, even within medical literature has been psycho-social, and there has been little critique of this approach. Much of the literature on IBS uses psycho-social assessment to imply or overtly to assert that psychological symptoms are present independently of the experience of symptoms of IBS and indeed precede them.

We can only speculate as to why the psycho-social explanation of IBS has become so ubiquitous. Other diseases with diarrhoea as a symptom have been associated with stress and psychological conditions and this may have become an accepted wisdom, taken for granted. Further, the move in sociological research away from single issue medical diagnoses may have been a factor.

Drossman et al. (1988) state that clinical findings in patients with IBS who seek health care do not explain the reported degree of distress and functional impairment, and that psychological assessment of IBS patients shows high prevalence of self reported stress, personality disorder and psychiatric diagnosis. From their multivariate study on patients with IBS, non-patients with IBS and what they call 'normal subjects' (Drossman et al., 1988, p. 701), they confirmed previous studies which found that IBS patients differ psychologically from IBS non-patients and normal subjects. They conclude from this that psychological factors influence how the illness is perceived and acted upon. In their systematic review Whitehead et al. (2002) reported that most of the studies that have assessed the overlap between IBS and psychiatric disorders show prevalence to be 90 per cent or more. They do, however, warn against drawing conclusions from this, as anxiety, depression, and somatization disorders are known to overlap in medical populations, but nevertheless conclude that most IBS patients have one or more psychiatric disorders. A problem with much of this research is that it is conducted with people who have received a diagnosis of IBS, and what cannot be assessed is whether they suffer more stress or psychiatric symptoms or whether the negative experience of the disease and of relationships with health professionals, as described by Dixon-Woods and Critchley (2000) below, leads to psychological changes in people. Comparing supposedly 'normal' controls with patient groups leads to assumptions about both groups that cannot be substantiated.

A study by Dixon-Woods and Critchley (2000) which uses qualitative methodology to investigate doctors' (GPs and gastroenterologists) and patients' views of IBS is an exception to the psycho-social body of work. The authors found that doctors often hold two definitions of IBS, a 'public' definition based on symptoms which reflected a textbook definition, and a 'private' definition that focused on the perceived characteristic of the typical IBS patient. This latter definition almost always referred to women. Doctors all felt that psychological factors were involved in the aetiology of IBS, but whereas some saw these as initiating and perpetuating it, describing patients as 'very stressed, obviously twitchy, quite neurotic' (Dixon-Woods and Critchley, 2000, p. 109), others viewed them as a consequence. A few doctors even felt that psychological factors had been implicated in IBS due to the failure of medical science to come up with a physiological explanation. Doctors also found IBS an unrewarding condition to treat, either because of the poor understanding of the disease and lack of effective treatments or because of the perception of the patients as problematic. They distinguished between 'good' patients who would accept the diagnosis given and accommodate it without making further demands for investigation or treatment, and 'bad' patients who resented the IBS label, and the psychological explanations of it.

For patients the significance of the symptoms was the interference with their daily lives, and although aware of the medical explanations would often reject them and look to other triggers for their symptoms, for example food intolerance. Patients were also aware of the negative labels, and saw themselves as a stigmatized and discredited group, who had been let down by the medical profession. As with endometriosis and back pain there is a discrepancy here between medical construction and patient experience of the condition.

Using the approaches taken for back pain and endometriosis and the social construction approach of Brown, a different interpretation and analysis of IBS can be formulated. Both IBS and endometriosis deal with bodily functions that have historical and cultural meanings. There are social norms that dictate how and with whom discussion on bowel function or menstruation takes place. This etiquette is breached by the person with IBS or endometriosis. Douglas (1966), in her seminal work on purity and danger, writes about leaky bodies, and how incontinence or flatulence is acceptable in babies, but one of the signs of maturity is the ability to maintain bodily integrity, that is to have control over the body and to dispose of bodily fluids in a culturally accepted way. People with IBS may breach this norm, and so symptoms have significance for patients beyond the biomedical categorization of them. For example, one woman wrote to a self help website:

> I feel dirty and horrible. I sometimes have to rush, but running can make it worse. Sometimes I have had to sit down on the pavement and wait for the cramps to go and then I can walk a bit more and get to the loo. Maybe adult nappies are the answer, but they won't disguise the smell will they? Oh it's too embarrassing to think about. (http://www.ibstales.com/diarrhea_tales_one.htm).

Bodily fluids are also associated with dirty work in the health and personal care sector, and the management of bowel function has little prestige in society (Denny, 2003). So patients may find that although IBS has great significance in their lives, and may dominate their social relationships, for a doctor it may be regarded as a trivial and low status activity.

In summary, IBS illustrates the tensions between patients and doctors over the diagnosis, interpretation and treatment of symptoms. The symptoms of flatulence, diarrhoea, bloating and constipation are commonly experienced in mild form in the general population, and are usually short lived and self limiting. For people with IBS the experience of these symptoms can severely affect their lives They are not, however, of interest to the medical profession as bodily fluids are associated with dirty work, and tend to be viewed as low status and unrewarding.

Summary and implications for nursing

In this chapter three themes have been identified for a sociological discussion of the conditions described which, it is argued, frequently elicit a negative response from the medical professions. These are problems surrounding diagnosis and treatment of symptoms, diseases and conditions that are not of interest to the medical profession, and conditions which are characterized by symptoms that are widespread in milder form in the general population. The label of 'heartsink' has been shown to be applied to the way health professionals feel about either the condition itself or the patient who experiences it.

From the three examples of low back pain, endometriosis and IBS we can draw together some common threads to develop a sociological understanding, which incorporates and builds upon the work of Waitzkin (1989), Bury (1991) and Brown (1995).

All of these diseases are characterized by common symptoms, most notably pain, that are frequently experienced by the general population, and the point at which these symptoms become more serious or unacceptable to the person experiencing them is a grey area. Within health services, the notion of when a commonly experienced symptom becomes serious enough to be regarded as a medical problem and not a variation of a 'normal' state is problematic, and may be a cause of tension between the patient and the health professionals they consult. The expectation of doctors in terms of diagnosis, treatment and outcome or resolution of symptoms is that diagnostic testing or some form of visualization will confirm disease, and that severity of disease will be consistent with presenting symptoms. When this does not occur, value judgements may well be made about 'appropriate' levels of pain or other symptoms associated with the observed degree of pathology, which does not equate with patient experience. In other words there is tension between the medical construction of disease and interpretation of presenting symptoms, and patient construction. For people living with a disease, these have to be located within the context of their lives, so that different facets have greater or lesser impact or significance on them.

These issues may be important in any doctor/patient relationship but for 'heartsink' patients there is the added complication that many of them suffer from contested conditions, such as those discussed in this chapter, with an uncertain disease trajectory and lack of effective treatments. They may well have spent years on the medical merry go round searching for an answer to their problems. Doctors see a snapshot of patients, who are trying to project an appropriate image during consultations, they do not see the impact of symptoms or disease on their lives. Encounters are controlled by the doctor who will ask questions designed to elicit the information s/he wants, rather than what the patient wants to tell them, and they are terminated at the behest of the doctor, often with no satisfactory outcome for the patient.

All of this leads us to a contradiction within this interpretation of events. When health professionals do move away from the biomedical model and use a psycho-social model to explain a patient's problems, this is often resisted and patients feel that any psychologizing of their symptoms is an implied character weakness. Despite dissatisfaction with their treatment within health services they still want an organic cause to be found for their problems, some pathology that will give them credibility in a way that a psychological label will not. Patients as well as health professionals are influenced by the perceived superiority of the biomedical model, and look to it for legitimation. Although they may not have faith in individual doctors, most people do have faith in a system of biomedicine They want the existing system to work for them in the same way that it works for those with uncontested diseases. They do not want to change the system.

Nurses, too, are grounded in the biomedical model of Western industrial health systems and rely on diagnostic tests and procedures in order to validate a patient's story. In order to move beyond this they need to understand the limitations of linear models of disease, and to accept that there may be alternative explanations. They need also to acknowledge that pain is not just a bio-psychological phenomenon, but an embodied, individual experience. In talking to people nurses are able to consider the patient's interpretation of what is happening to them, which may not be consistent with the results of biomedical procedures. It is only by listening to patient experience that nurses will come to know the significance a disease has on their lives. What is of major importance to them may be considered by health professionals to be trivial, and not of any clinical interest. In order for 'heartsink' patients to lose their pejorative label more credibility needs to be given to what they tell health professionals, even when this seems to contradict the perceived superiority of objective measurement.

References

Atkinson P., 'The reproduction of medical knowledge', in R. Dingwall, C. Heath, M. Reid and M. Stacey, *Health Care and Health Knowledge* (London: Croom Helm, 1977).

Balint M., *The Doctor, His Patient and the Illness* (London: Pitman, 1957).

Ballard K., K. Lowton and J. Wright, 'What's the delay? A qualitative study of women's experiences of reaching a diagnosis of endometriosis', *Fertility and Sterility*, 86 (2006) 1296–1301.

Bendelow G., 'Pain perceptions, gender and emotion', *Sociology of Health and Illness*, 15 (1993) 273–294.

Brown P., 'Naming and framing: the social construction of diagnosis and illness', *Journal of Health and Social Behaviour,* Extra issue (1995) 34–52.

Bury M., 'The sociology of chronic illness: a review', *Sociology of Health and Illness*, 13 (1991) 451–468.

Butler C.C., and M. Evans, 'The heartsink patient revisited', *British Journal of General Practice*, 49 (1999) 230–233.

Cox H., L. Henderson, N. Andersen et al., 'Focus group study of endometriosis: struggle, loss and the medical merry-go-round', *International Journal of Nursing Practice*, 9 (2003) 2–9.

Denny E., 'The class context of nursing', in M. Miers (ed.), *Class, Inequalities and Nursing Practice* (Basingstoke: Palgrave, 2003).

Denny E., 'Women's experience of endometriosis' *Journal of Advanced Nursing*, 46 (2004b) 641–648.

Denny E., ' "You are one of the unlucky ones" Delay in diagnosis of endometriosis', *Diversity in Health and Social Care*, 1: 1 (2004a) 39–44.

Denny E., C.H. Mann, 'Endometriosis and the primary care consultation', *European Journal of Obstetrics & Gynaecology and Reproductive Health Care*, 139 (2008) 111–115.

Dixon-Woods M., and S. Critchley 'Medical and lay views of irritable bowel syndrome', *Family Practice*, 17 (2000) 108–113.

Douglas M., *Purity and Danger* (London: Routledge, 1966).

Drossman D.A., D.C. McKee, R.S. Sandler, M. Mitchell, E.M. Cramer, B.C. Lowman, A.L. Burger, 'Psychosocial factors in the irritable bowel syndrome', *Gastroenterology*, 95 (1988) 701–708.

Fox R., 'Medical uncertainty revisited', in G.L. Albrecht, R. Fitzpatrick, S.C.Scrimshaw (eds) *The Handbook of Social Studies in Health and Medicine* (London: Sage, 2000).

Glenton C., 'Chronic back pain sufferers – striving for the sick role', *Social Science and Medicine*, 57 (2003) 2243–2252.

Hadfield R., H. Mardon, D. Barlow, S. Kennedy, 'Delay in the diagnosis of endometriosis: a survey of women from the USA and the UK', *Human Reproduction*, 11 (1996) 878–880.

Huntington A., G.A. Gilmour, 'A life shaped by pain: women and endometriosis', *Journal of Advanced Nursing*, 14 (2005) 1124–1132.

Hydén L., 'Illness and narrative', *Sociology of Health and Illness*, 19 (1997) 48–69.

Illich I., *Medical Nemesis. The Expropriation of Health* (New York: Random House, 1976).

Illingworth R.S., 'Why irritated?', *Archives of Diseases in Childhood*, 63 (1988) 567–568.

Jones G., C. Jenkinson, S. Kennedy, 'The impact of endometriosis on quality of life: a qualitative analysis', *Journal of Psychosomatic Obstetrics and Gynaecology*, 25 (2004) 123–133.

Lemaire G.S., 'More than just menstrual cramps: Symptoms and uncertainty among women with endometriosis', *Journal of Obstetrics, Gynaecology and Neonatal Nursing*, 33 (2004) 71–79.

Mantle H., 'Every part of my body hurt', *Society Guardian* (2004) Available from http://society.guardian.co.uk/health/story/0,7890, 1232986,00.html (last accessed 9 December2007.

May C., G. Allison A. Chapple, C. Chew-Graham, C. Dixon, L. Gask et al., 'Framing the doctor patient relationship in chronic illness: A comparative study of general practitioners' accounts', *Sociology of Health and Illness*, 26 (2004) 135–158.

Miller J., and D. Timpson, 'Exploring the experience of partners who live with a chronic low back pain sufferer', *Health and Social Care in the Community*, 12: 1 (2004) 34–42.

O'Dowd T.C., 'Five years of heartsink patients in general practice', *British Medical Journal*, 297 (1988) 528–530.

Rhodes L.A., C.A. McPhillips-Tangum, C. Markham and R. Klenk, 'The power of the visible: the meaning of diagnostic tests in chronic back pain', in S. Nettleton and U. Gustafsson (eds) *The Sociology of Health and Illness Reader* (Cambridge: Polity, 2002).

Talley N.J., P.M. Boyce, M. Jones, 'Predictors of health care seeking for irritable bowel syndrome: a population based study', *Gut*, 41 (1997) 394–398.

Waitzkin H., 'A critical theory of medical discourse: ideology, social control, and the processing of social context in medical encounters', *Journal of Health and Social Behaviour*, 30 (1989) 220–239.

Whitehead W.E., O. Palsson, K.R. Jones, 'Systematic review of the comorbidity of irritable bowel syndrome with other disorders: what are the causes and implications?', *Gastroenterology*, 122 (2002) 1140–1156.

Williams S.J., *Medicine and the Body* (London, Sage 2003).

Concluding reflections

Elaine Denny and Sarah Earle

Most of us are living longer lives and yet we are unlikely to live these extra years in perfect health. Although there is no 'cure' for the majority of long-term conditions, many of them can be managed successfully for years – if not indefinitely. However, the personal costs of living with a long-term condition can be high, affecting both physical and mental health as well as overall feelings of wellbeing. The economic and social costs of managing these conditions (including the costs of health and social care, loss of earnings, and so on) are also enormous.

Whilst this book is not comprehensive, and no book of this kind could hope to be so, we have attempted to bring together key sociological work in the area of long-term conditions and to emphasize those conditions which pose some of the most serious threats to morbidity and mortality today and in the future. The book begins by providing a brief overview of sociological theory, drawing on bodies of knowledge that focus on sickness, chronic illness, disability and the body. Early writers in the genre chose to focus on these conditions at a time when the emphasis of health research and policy was acute illness. They drew attention to the problems facing those who often suffered in silence with illness for which there was no cure, and the problems faced by those affected – patients, families, and carers. They recognized the heavy burden that living with long term illness placed on people and demonstrated this by conducting research on the experience of patients and their carers, gaining insight into their worlds. Capturing this experience provided an understanding that was not apparent in the quantitative research on diagnosis, treatments and clinical outcomes.

Part I also explores the policy process and discussed the extent to which the epidemiological explosion of chronic illness comprises a policy problem. The importance of policy-making in health care is increasingly at the forefront of public debate. For example, it is only necessary to briefly scan the weekly newspapers or news channels to come across dozens of articles on the subject (e.g., see Benjamin, 2007; Meikle, 2008; Pisani, 2008). The final chapter in Part I focuses on research methods, methodology and epistemology in relation to the wide ranging research which concerns nurses working with people who have long-term conditions. And, as the author of this chapter writes,

> People new to research may be forgiven for thinking that this chapter is one to skip over before getting to the more interesting ones... But, social researchers (and physical scientists and health researchers), need to be clear about their motivations for research, their methods of data collection and how the research process affects the research product. (Letherby, this volume, p. 56).

Needless to say that most practitioners are aware of the importance of research for practice, and although not all nurses are directly involved in the research process, the products of research are of vital importance to everyday policy and practice in the care of people with long-term conditions.

Sociological health research underpins all of the chapters presented in Part II of the book. Such research encompasses small-scale qualitative studies which explore the experiences of people living with long-term conditions, as well as surveys and health services evaluations (Bowling, 2002). Indeed, in some of the chapters presented here, authors have drawn on their own empirical work to explore the sociology of long-term conditions. For example, in Chapter 5, Lesley Lockyer draws on her qualitative study of professional and lay accounts of Coronary Heart Disease (CHD), examining the gendered experiences of this long-term condition. Similarly, in Chapter 7, Jonathan Tritter discusses the findings of a research project which explored patients' understandings and perceptions of living with a range of cancers.

All of the chapters in this book are strongly underpinned by both classic and contemporary sociological theory and research. Whilst experiences of living with a long-term condition are unique, there are also commonalities in experience.

Some of these commonalities and shared themes are expressed throughout this book.

The importance of listening to, understanding, and acting upon, the perspectives of patients and clients is increasingly being recognized within nursing, and in health (and social care) more generally. For example, the *Health in Partnership* research programme concluded that: 'The involvement of patients, carers and the public in health decision-making is at the heart of the modernisation of the National Health Service (NHS)... Patient involvement increases patient satisfaction ... Patients feel involved in their care when they are treated as equal partners, listened to and properly informed' (DH, 2004, p. 2).

Indeed the principle of user involvement is central to the *Expert Patient Programme* (www.expertpatients.co.uk) and other similar schemes. Of course whilst there are considerable barriers to the involvement of patients and the public in health research, service delivery and development (Branfield and Beresford, 2006), and the concept is not without its critics (Cowden and Singh, 2007; Fudge, Wolfe and McKevitt, 2008; Smith et al., 2008), certain sociological approaches to the study of long-term conditions play an important role in promoting an understanding of the patients' perspective. Interpretive sociology, for example, seeks to understand chronic illness by exploring the experiences of those living with such a condition. Much of this interpretive work has focused on how people living with a long-term condition – such as epilepsy or psoriasis – describe the difficulties they face and how they cope with them (e.g., see Roth, 1963; Jobling, 1988). The concept of biographical disruption has also been influential in understanding how people experience living with a long-term condition (see Bury, 1982, 1991) and narrative approaches attempt to explore the way that individuals use 'illness narratives' to explain their experience of chronic illness within the context of their own personal biography. Indeed, writing within this sociological perspective, Hydén (1997, p. 49) suggests that illness narratives give a 'voice to suffering'.

All of the chapters in Part II of this book give voice to the perspectives of people who live with a long-term condition and squarely focus on their needs and experiences. Chapter 4, by Tom Heller, draws on the work of Odencrants, Ehnfors and

Grobe (2005) who consider the experiences of people with Chronic Obstructive Pulmonary Disease (COPD) and their relationship to food. This chapter also draws on the work of Guthrie, Hill and Muers (2001) who report the fear and restrictions that continual breathlessness can bring about in people living with COPD. In Lesley Lockyer's chapter on CHD attention focuses on the importance of 'lay accounts' and on what these can reveal about health and illness (see Chapter 5). Here, Lockyer argues that whilst practitioners often focus on the acute and dramatic consequences of CHD, lay accounts reveal that patients are most concerned with the chronic aspects of this condition. In Chapter 6, Cathy E. Lloyd and T. Chas Skinner review policy and practice in diabetes care, highlighting the significance of an 'empowerment approach' to care which encourages the involvement of people with diabetes in determining local health services and priorities. However, no-where is the significance of giving voice to people who live with chronic illness more poignant than in the chapter by Pauline Savy (see Chapter 9). This chapter focuses on the experiences of people who suffer from dementia and here, drawing on the concepts of 'witness' and 'duty', (Frank, 1995) Savy argues that nurses play an important role in giving voice to those who suffer from this heartbreaking condition.

The concept of stigma is also an important recurring theme throughout this book. Originally attributable to the work of sociologist Erving Goffman (1963), but widely adopted in both sociological and other research, stigma can manifest as either a 'discrediting' or a 'discreditable' attribute. According to Goffman, stigma can also be experienced as either 'felt' or 'enacted' (see Fraser and Treloar, 2006) and 'courtesy stigma' refers to the impact of stigma on friends and family (e.g., see Corrigan and Miller, 2004). The concept of stigma is useful in gaining a deeper understanding of the experiences of those living with a long-term condition and the consequences of this for them and those around them.

Many of the chapters in this book explore the stigma of living with chronic illness. For example, in Chapter 8 Erica Richardson examines the experiences of People Living with HIV/AIDS (PLWHA) arguing that those living with this treatable – but incurable – condition, 'are feared and highly stigmatized' (this volume, p. 169). Richardson concludes by arguing that nurses are well placed to challenge the stigma experienced by PLWHA but that the provision of holistic care requires an understanding of how HIV has been stigmatized and what this actually means in practice. Similarly, Chapter 12 explores the experiences of 'heartsink' patients – or rather – those patients who have a long-term condition which is causing pain and distress but for which either no cause can be found or no treatment has been successful (O'Dowd, 1988). In this chapter, Elaine Denny discusses the perspectives of those living with chronic back pain, endometriosis and Irritable Bowel Syndrome (IBS) to explore the way in which such individuals are stigmatized and discredited. In Chapter 11, Sarah Earle focuses on experiences of obesity and challenges nurses to reflect on their own personal beliefs and actions. Drawing on empirical work in this field, Earle shows how people labelled as overweight and obese are shamed and blamed for their condition whilst also experiencing discrimination in access to health care (see Wills et al., 2006 and Carryer, 2007).

Nurses are at the forefront of providing care to the many people who live with one, or more, long-term conditions. Nurse specialists, for example, provide invaluable support to enable those living with a long-term condition to manage their symptoms and treatment. Nurse-led services are also central to the public health work which takes place in the prevention of long term ill-health. However, clinical expertise and experience alone are insufficient in the drive to provide good quality health care. We have chosen to develop this book because we believe that a sociological imagination can assist nurses in providing care for people with long-term conditions. We hope that you have enjoyed using this book, that it has stimulated your sociological imagination and made a contribution to your knowledge and understanding in this field.

References

Benjamin A., 'Hospital parking "a stealth tax on illness"', *The Guardian*, Wednesday 21 March 2007.

Bowling A., *Research Methods in Health*, 2nd edn (Buckingham: Open University Press, 2002).

Branfield F., and P. Beresford with E.J. Andres, P. Chambers, P. Staddon, G. Wise and B. Williams-Findlay, *Making User Involvement Work: Supporting Service User Networking and Knowledge* (York: Joseph Rowntree Foundation, 2006).

Bury M., 'Chronic illness as biographical disruption', *Sociology of Health & Illness*, 4: 2 (1982) 167–182.

Bury M., 'The sociology of chronic illness', *Sociology of Health & Illness*, 13: 4 (1991) 263–285.

Carryer J., 'Embodied largeness: a significant women's health issue', *Nursing Inquiry*, 8: 2 (2001) 90–97.

Corrigan P.W., and F.E. Miller, 'Shame, blame and contamination: A review of the impact of mental illness stigma on family members', *Journal of Mental Health*, 13: 6 (2004), 537–548.

Cowden S., and G. Singh, 'The "user": friend, foe or fetish? A critical exploration of user involvement in health and social care', *Critical Social Policy*, 27: 1 (2007) 5–23.

Department of Health/Christine Farrell (DH) *Patient and Public Involvement in Health: The Evidence for Policy Implementation*. (London: DH, 2004).

Expert Patient Programme, www.expertpatient.co.uk (online) (last accessed 13 May 2008).

Frank A., *The Wounded Storyteller: Body, Illness and Ethics* (Chicago: University of Chicago Press, 1995).

Fraser S., and C. Treloar, ' "Spoiled identity" in hepatitis C infection: The binary logic of despair', *Critical Public Health*, 16: 2 (2006) 99–110.

Fudge N., C.D.A. Wolfe and C. McKevitt, 'Assessing the promise of user involvement in health service development: ethnographic study', *British Medical Journal*, 336: 7639 (2008) 313–317.

Goffman E., *Stigma: Notes on the Management of a Spoiled Identity* (London: Penguin Books, 1963).

Guthrie S., K. Hill and M. Muers, 'Living with severe COPD. A qualitative exploration of the experience of patients in Leeds', *Respiratory Medicine*, 95 (2001) 196–204.

Hydén L.C., 'Illness and narrative', *Sociology of Health and Illness*, 19: 1 (1997) 48–69.

Jobling R., 'The experience of psoriasis under treatment', in R. Anderson and M. Bury (eds) *Living with Chronic Illness: The Experience of Patients and their Families* (London: Unwin Hyman, 1988).

Meikle J., 'Appeal court ruling gives hope to NHS Alzheimer's patients denied drugs', *The Guardian*, Friday 2 May 2008, http://www.guardian.co.uk/society/2008/may/02/health. mentalhealth (last accessed 12 September 2008).

Odencrants S., M. Ehnfors and S. Grobe, 'Living with chronic obstructive pulmonary disease: Part 1. Stuggling with meal-related situations: experiences among persons with COPD', *Scandinavian Journal of Caring Sciences*, 19 (2005) 230–239.

O'Dowd T.C., 'Five years of heartsink patients in general practice', *British Medical Journal*, 297 (1988) 528–530.

Pisani E., 'The unspoken truth about Aids', *The Sunday Times*, 4 May 2008.

Roth J.A., *Timetables: Structuring the Passage of Time in Hospital Treatment and Other Careers* (Indianapolis: Bobbs Merrill, 1963).

Smith E., F. Ross, S. Donovan, J. Manthorpe, S. Brearley, J. Sitzia and P. Beresford, 'Service user involvement in nursing, midwifery and health visiting research: A review of evidence and practice', *International Journal of Nursing Studies*, 45: 2 (2008) 298–315.

Wills W., K. Backett-Milburn, S. Gregory and J. Lawton, ' "Young teenagers" perceptions of their own and others' bodies: A qualitative study of obese, overweight and "normal" weight young people in Scotland', *Social Science & Medicine*, 62 (2006) 396–406.

Index